MW00511751

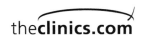

HAND CLINICS

Contemporary Issues Related to Management of the Upper Limb in Tetraplegia

GUEST EDITORS
Mary Jane Mulcahey, PhD, OTR/L
Albert A. Weiss, MD, MBA

May 2008 • Volume 24 • Number 2

SAUNDERS

An Imprint of Elsevier, Inc.
PHILADELPHIA   LONDON   TORONTO   MONTREAL   SYDNEY   TOKYO

W.B. SAUNDERS COMPANY

A Division of Elsevier Inc.

1600 John F. Kennedy Blvd. • Suite 1800 • Philadelphia, Pennsylvania 19103

http://www.theclinics.com

HAND CLINICS
May 2008
Editor: Debora Dellapena

Volume 24, Number 2
ISSN 0749-0712
ISBN-13: 978-1-4160-5815-1
ISBN-10: 1-4160-5815-X

Copyright © 2008 by Elsevier Inc. All rights reserved. No part of this publication may be reproduced or transmitted in any form or by any means, electronic or mechanical, including photocopy, recording, or any information retrieval system, without written permission from the publisher.

Single photocopies of single articles may be made for personal use as allowed by national copyright laws. Permission of the publisher and payment of a fee is required for all other photocopying, including multiple or systematic copying, copying for advertising or promotional purposes, resale, and all forms of document delivery. Special rates are available for educational institutions that wish to make photocopies for non-profit educational classroom use. Permissions may be sought directly from Elsevier's Rights Department in Philadelphia, PA, USA: phone: (+1) 215 239 3804, fax: (+1) 215 239 3805, e-mail: healthpermissions@elsevier.com. Requests may also be completed on-line via the Elsevier homepage (http://www.elsevier.com/locate/permissions). In the USA, users may clear permissions and make payments through the Copyright Clearance Center, Inc., 222 Rosewood Drive, Danvers, MA 01923, USA; phone: (978) 750-8400; fax: (978) 750-4744, and in the UK through the Copyright Licensing Agency Rapid Clearance Service (CLARCS), 90 Tottenham Court Road, London W1P 0LP, UK; phone: (+44) 171 436 5931; fax: (+44) 171 436 3986. Others countries may have a local reprographic rights agency for payments.

The ideas and opinions expressed in *Hand Clinics* do not necessarily reflect those of the Publisher. The Publisher does not assume any responsibility for any injury and/or damage to persons or property arising out of or related to any use of the material contained in this periodical. The reader is advised to check the appropriate medical literature and the product information provided by the manufacturer of each drug to be administered to verify the dosage, the method and duration of administration, or contraindications. It is the responsibility of the treating physician or other health care professional, relying on independent experience and knowledge of the patient, to determine drug dosages and the best treatment for the patient. Mention of any product in this issue should not be construed as endorsement by the contributors, editors, or the Publisher of the product or manufacturers' claims.

Hand Clinics (ISSN 0749-0712) is published quarterly by Elsevier Inc., 360 Park Avenue South, New York, NY 10010-1710. Months of publication are February, May, August, and November. Business and Editorial Offices: 1600 John F. Kennedy Blvd., Suite 1800, Philadelphia, PA 19103-2899. Customer Service Office: 6277 Sea Harbor Drive, Orlando, FL 32887-4800. Periodicals postage paid at New York, NY, and additional mailing offices. Subscription price is $261.00 per year (U.S. individuals), $405.00 per year (U.S. institutions), $133.00 per year (US students), $297.00 per year (Canadian individuals), $454.00 per year (Canadian institutions), $164.00 (Canadian students), $333.00 per year (international individuals), $454.00 per year (international institutions), and $164.00 per year (international students). Foreign air speed delivery is included in all *Clinics* subscription prices. All prices are subject to change without notice. POSTMASTER: Send address changes to *Hand Clinics*, Elsevier Periodicals Customer Service, 6277 Sea Harbor Drive, Orlando, FL 32887-4800. Customer Service: 1-800-654-2452 (US). From outside the United States, call 1-407-563-6020. Fax: 1-407-363-9661. E-mail: JournalsCustomerService-usa@elsevier.com.

Reprints. For copies of 100 or more, of articles in this publication, please contact the Commercial Rights Department, Elsevier Inc., 360 Park Avenue South, New York, NY 10010-1710. Tel: (212) 633-3813, Fax: (212) 462-1935, e-mail: reprints@elsevier.com.

Hand Clinics is covered in *Index Medicus, Current Contents/Clinical Medicine, EMBASE/Excerpta Medica,* and *ISI/BIOMED.*

Printed in the United States of America.

GUEST EDITORS

MARY JANE MULCAHEY, PhD, OTR/L, Director of Rehabilitation Services and Clinical Research, Shriners Hospital for Children, Philadelphia, Pennsylvania

ALBERT A. WEISS, MD, MBA, Associate Professor of Orthopedic Surgery, Department of Orthopedic Surgery, Temple University School of Medicine; Consulting Surgeon, Shriners Hospital for Children, Philadelphia, Pennsylvania

CONTRIBUTORS

ANNE M. BRYDEN, OTR/L, Research Occupational Therapist, The Cleveland Functional Electrical Stimulation Center, MetroHealth Medical Center, Cleveland, Ohio

KEVIN C. CHUNG, MD, MS, Professor of Surgery, Section of Plastic Surgery, Department of Surgery, University of Michigan Health System, Ann Arbor, Michigan

SANDRA J. CONNOLLY, BHScOT, OT Reg (Ont), St. Joseph's Health Care London, Parkwood Hospital, London, Ontario, Canada

JENNIFER A. DUNN, Dip PT, MPhil, Physiotherapy Department, Burwood Spinal Unit, Christchurch, New Zealand

VINCENT R. HENTZ, MD, Professor of Surgery and Orthopaedic Surgery (by Courtesy), Stanford University School of Medicine; Consulting Surgeon, Spinal Cord Injury Unit, Veteran Affairs Palo Alto Health Care System; Stanford University Medical Center, Palo Alto, California

SCOTT H. KOZIN, MD, Associate Professor, Department of Orthopaedic Surgery, Temple University; Director, Pediatric Hand and Upper Extremity Center of Excellence, Shriners Hospitals for Children, Philadelphia, Pennsylvania

CAROLINE LECLERCQ, MD, Hand Surgeon and Consultant, Institut de la Main, Clinique Jouvenet; Coubert Rehabilitation Center; Ancien Chef de Clinique Hôpitaux de Paris; Consultant, Centre de Rééducation Neurologique et Fonctionelle, Coubert, France

MARY JANE MULCAHEY, PhD, OTR/L, Director of Rehabilitation Services and Clinical Research, Shriners Hospitals for Children, Philadelphia, Pennsylvania

ALASTAIR G. ROTHWELL, ONZM, MB, ChM, FRACS, Burwood Spinal Unit; Professor, Department of Orthopaedic Surgery and Musculoskeletal Medicine, University of Otago, Christchurch School of Medicine and Health Sciences, Christchurch, New Zealand

K. ANNE SINNOTT, Dip PT, MPhty, Burwood Spinal Unit; Department of Orthopaedic Surgery and Musculoskeletal Medicine, University of Otago, Christchurch School of Medicine and Health Sciences, Christchurch, New Zealand

LEE SQUITIERI, BS, Medical Student, The University of Michigan Medical School, Ann Arbor, Michigan

ALBERT A. WEISS, MD, MBA, Associate Professor of Orthopedic Surgery, Department of Orthopedic Surgery, Temple University School of Medicine; Consulting Surgeon, Shriners Hospital for Children, Philadelphia, Pennsylvania

CONTENTS

Dedication   ix
Alastair G. Rothwell

Preface   xi
Mary Jane Mulcahey and Albert A. Weiss

Contemporary Trends in Management of the Upper Limb in Tetraplegia:
A Multinational Perspective   157
Albert A. Weiss

> The 2007 Meeting on Upper Limb in Tetraplegia in Philadelphia provided an opportunity to explore individual and regional differences in surgeons' preferences in tetraplegic upper limb reconstruction. Reports were heard from New Zealand, Canada, Asia, Australia, and Europe. Most presenters attempted to gather data from across their regions. Each reporter made a sincere effort to identify the spectrum of the quality of the data, as well as the opportunities for regional progress. Completeness of reports varied, depending on sophistication of the available data collection agencies. Notwithstanding limitations and omissions, the commonalities and differences revealed in those reports were enlightening and provide opportunities for fruitful study. This article represents a compilation of presentations on regional trends by invited participants.

Measurement Issues Related to Upper Limb Interventions in Persons
Who Have Tetraplegia   161
Jennifer A. Dunn, K. Anne Sinnott, Anne M. Bryden, Sandra J. Connolly,
and Alastair G. Rothwell

> Measurement of upper limb function in persons with tetraplegia poses significant issues for clinicians and researchers. It is crucial that measures detect the small but significant improvements in hand function that may or may not occur as a result of our interventions. Before determining how we measure changes from upper limb interventions, we must establish what outcomes are of greatest interest, and for whom. Many issues have an impact on both the measurement and interpretative process.

Current Utilization of Reconstructive Upper Limb Surgery in Tetraplegia   169
Lee Squitieri and Kevin C. Chung

> Despite improved surgical techniques and postoperative management protocols for tetraplegic patients undergoing upper extremity functional reconstruction, recent studies

have shown that these procedures are profoundly underutilized in the United States. The complex disabilities of tetraplegic patients limit their ability to independently obtain treatment information and travel to medical destinations to receive reconstructive procedures, thus making them a vulnerable patient population susceptible to physician influence regarding treatment decisions. Based on the results of previous research, we believe that increased collaboration among treating physician specialties will enhance patient access to surgical reconstruction.

The Management of the Upper Limb in Incomplete Lesions of the Cervical Spinal Cord   175
Vincent R. Hentz and Caroline Leclercq

Patients with incomplete cervical spinal cord injuries present unique challenges for the reconstructive surgeon. For example, their patterns of injury don't easily fit into the International Classification system familiar to surgeons; they don't lend themselves to a "recipe" approach to surgical decision-making; and they frequently have developed upper limb deformities that must be addressed before any consideration is made for functional surgery. Meanwhile, little has been published regarding surgery for these patients. This article summarizes issues related to evaluating and planning surgical procedures for the upper limb in incomplete lesions of the cervical spinal cord.

Reconstruction of Elbow Extension   185
Caroline Leclercq, Vincent R. Hentz, Scott H. Kozin, and Mary Jane Mulcahey

The loss of elbow extension power is particularly disabling for the nonambulatory patient. Reconstruction of elbow extension can be performed by a deltoid to triceps transfer or by a biceps to triceps transfer provides the most satisfying reconstruction for patients. Although the overall time for rehabilitation can be lengthy, the functional gain is substantial, predictable, and easily appreciated by the patient. Furthermore, the risks to residual preoperative function are practically nil.

Pediatric Onset Spinal Cord Injury: Implications on Management of the Upper Limb in Tetraplegia   203
Scott H. Kozin

This article focuses on the pediatric upper limb after spinal cord injury and highlights the obstacles during reconstruction.

Index   215

FORTHCOMING ISSUES

August 2008

Thumb Arthritis
Tamara D. Rozental, MD, *Guest Editor*

November 2008

Nerve Transfers
Susan MacKinnon, MD, and
Christine Novak, PT, MSc, PhD, *Guest Editors*

February 2009

Evidence-Based Practice
Robert M. Szabo, MD, and
Joy C. MacDermid, BScPT, PhD, *Guest Editors*

RECENT ISSUES

February 2008

Acute and Chronic Elbow Instability
Scott G. Edwards, MD, *Guest Editor*

November 2007

Humerus Fractures
Scott P. Steinmann, MD, *Guest Editor*

August 2007

The Ulnar Nerve
Dan A. Zlotolow, MD, and
Vincent D. Pellegrini, Jr, MD, *Guest Editors*

THE CLINICS ARE NOW AVAILABLE ONLINE!

Access your subscription at
www.theclinics.com

ELSEVIER
SAUNDERS

Hand Clin 24 (2008) ix–x

HAND
CLINICS

Dedication

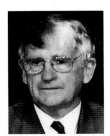

Alan Maxwell Clarke
(1932–2007)

On January 21, 2007, New Zealand lost Alan Maxwell Clarke, who was a wonderful ambassador for the independent living cause. Possessing a powerful intellect and an incredibly strong will, Alan doggedly pursued his campaign for people living with disability to take ownership and control of their individual destinies and escape the clutches of well meaning health professionals who insisted the management of the disabled was their domain. One of his catch cries was that health professionals should be "on tap" and not "on top".

Born in 1932 to a surgeon father and a nurse mother, Alan graduated from the Otago Medical School, New Zealand in 1956. Five years later he qualified as a surgeon, and after 2 years in Glasgow as a general surgical fellow, he returned to New Zealand in 1964 as a consultant surgeon. Alan became a prominent international contributor, particularly in the bowel cancer field, and in 1970 at only 38 years old, he was appointed professor of surgery at the University of Otago. He was forced to give up this position 15 years later following major surgery for bladder cancer.

In 1986 he was appointed Dean of the Christchurch School of Medicine and Health Sciences, and during his tenure, he controversially banned lectures for medical students, favoring instead a culture of self directed learning. The Christchurch medical students subsequently outperformed their peers from other New Zealand medical schools. This successful experiment in self directed learning sowed the seeds of Alan's later advocacy of self directed living and learning in the years to come.

On April 14, 1991 Alan fell from his roof and became paraplegic. He was admitted to the Burwood Spinal Unit and set new standards in patient noncompliance, because he argued, debated, and disagreed on nearly every aspect of his rehabilitation process. A watershed experience occurred early in his rehabilitation when he asked the night nurse to pass him his water jug. "Do it your bloody self" was the abrupt reply, and once over the initial shock of that response, Alan realized how easy it could be to fall into the dependency trap. Furthermore, the rehabilitation experience further enhanced his view that many aspects of the process are, in themselves, disabling, and that people consequently learn dependency. He also discovered that rehabilitation is a process of self learning and not a medical process. Alan left the Burwood Spinal Unit in record time and returned to his deanship of the Otago Medical School within 4 months of his injury. His rehabilitation experiences and his experience learning to live in a wheelchair in the outside world reinforced that the currently practiced processes of rehabilitation had to be changed radically. In 1994 he resigned from the deanship and successfully applied for the clinical director position at the Burwood Spinal

0749-0712/08/$ - see front matter © 2008 Elsevier Inc. All rights reserved.
doi:10.1016/j.hcl.2008.01.002

Unit. During his tenure, he established the New Zealand Spinal Trust as the vehicle for assisting disabled people to take charge of their rehabilitation. One of its key objectives is to encourage and foster a philosophy of rehabilitation that focuses on the full attainment of personal potential and ability with personal control and responsibility.

In 10 short years the New Zealand Spinal Trust established the New Zealand-wide spinal network through which all spinal cord injured persons and families can freely communicate; worked with the New Zealand Rugby Football Union to dramatically reduce scrum related neck injuries; established the Kaleidoscope Vocational Rehabilitation Programme, which facilitates the attainment of work and financial independence for spinal cord injured persons; and built the unique Alan Bean Centre, resourced to provide the highest quality information for spinal cord injured and other disabled people, which will help them take charge of their rehabilitation. Alan also spearheaded the development of New Zealand-wide service guidelines for the total lifelong management of spinal cord injured persons, which emphasized rehabilitation in terms of diversity, ability, and participation rather than deficit, disability, and function.

In the late 1990's Alan embraced the concept of the independent living paradigm in which patients are consumers, are in charge, are the decision makers, are chairmen of the board, or (with regard to spinal cord injured persons) are spinal ferraris. Health professionals are staff in charge of the clinical task and keep the spinal ferraris in tip top race condition, but they most definitely do not tell them where and how to drive.

The culmination of all of Alan's thinking and advocacy led to the development of the Burwood Academy of Independent Living, which was aimed at establishing a learning academy based on the principals of the independent living paradigm. Alan was the patron of the academy to ensure that these principals were fully implemented. At the time of his sudden death, Alan was writing a book that embodied the principals of the independent living paradigm, freely illustrated with personal stories.

In 1996 the Queen of England bestowed on Alan the Companion of the Most Excellent Order of St Michael and St George for services to medicine and surgery.

Throughout his years as a dedicated advocate for the spinal cord injured person, Alan was also strongly supportive of the upper limb surgery service at the Burwood Spinal Unit. He likened the staff to engineers charged with providing maximum upper limb function in order to maximize the ferrari performance! On a number of occasions he facilitated visits of overseas experts, raised money for some of the more expensive upper limb procedures, and enabled local staff to visit centers overseas.

At the 8th International Meeting of Upper Limb Surgery for Tetraplegia, he delivered the Keynote Opening Address based on the independent living paradigm despite having had life threatening major abdominal surgery a few weeks earlier. His speech made a big impact on those present.

Alan's legacy is huge and cannot be condensed into a few words, but his message to all readers would be to embrace the independent living paradigm, the characteristics of which are:

I am a person, consumer or a customer
My problems are my undue reliance on professionals and family, environmental barriers, and discrimination
My solutions are peer support, self help (being in charge), and access to services that meet my needs
I am accountable and responsible to myself
The outcomes I seek are to be in charge of my life, to live independently with disability, to be fulfilled, and to be financially secure.

Alan was the living embodiment of the independent living paradigm and his "Do it your bloody self" philosophy.

Alastair G. Rothwell, ONZM, MB,
ChM, FRACS
*Department of Orthopaedic Surgery
and Musculoskeletal Medicine
University of Otago
Christchurch School of Medicine
and Health Sciences
P.O. Box 4710
Christchurch, New Zealand*

E-mail address: alastairrothwell@chmeds.ac.nz

ELSEVIER
SAUNDERS

Hand Clin 24 (2008) xi

HAND
CLINICS

Preface

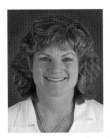 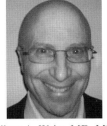

Mary Jane Mulcahey, PhD, OTR\L   Albert A. Weiss, MD, MBA
Guest Editors

This is the second issue of *Hand Clinics* that is dedicated entirely to research and clinical interventions for restoration of hand and arm function in people who have tetraplegia. This issue is based largely on the recent International Meeting on Upper Limb in Tetraplegia that was held in Philadelphia in September 2007 for approximately 150 interested clinicians.

As a direct result of their collaboration, surgical techniques and assistive technologies for improved upper limb function have advanced greatly—giving people who have spinal cord injury monumentally improved capabilities for engagement in work, self care, and leisure. Part of the meeting focused on the study of meaningful outcomes–those that are important to people who have tetraplegia–enabling researchers and clinicians to better meet the expectations of those receiving upper limb care.

This issue of *Hand Clinics* addresses contemporary principles related to the upper limb in tetraplegia: outcomes, assessments, and measurement issues; surgical technique and rehabilitation of elbow extension transfers; and management of the hand of persons who have incomplete injuries. In addition, international participants present a summary of contemporary perspectives. Lastly, and with much enthusiasm, a discussion of shoulder modeling is introduced as an important area of consideration when managing the upper limb of persons who have spinal cord injury.

Mary Jane Mulcahey, PhD, OTR/L
Albert A. Weiss, MD, MBA
Shriners Hospital for Children
3551 North Broad Street
Philadelphia, PA 19140, USA

E-mail addresses: mmulcahey@shrinenet.org;
bertieweiss@hotmail.com

0749-0712/08/$ - see front matter © 2008 Elsevier Inc. All rights reserved.
doi:10.1016/j.hcl.2008.02.002

Contemporary Trends in Management of the Upper Limb in Tetraplegia: A Multinational Perspective

Albert A. Weiss, MD, MBA[a,b,*]

[a]*Department of Orthopedic Surgery, Temple University School of Medicine, 3401 North Broad Street, 6th Floor, Philadelphia, PA 19140, USA*
[b]*Shriners Hospital for Children, 3551 North Broad Street, Philadelphia, PA 19140, USA*

This article represents a compilation of presentations on regional trends by invited participants of the 2007 Meeting on Upper Limb in Tetraplegia in Philadelphia [1]. Representatives of all geographic regions were invited, and many provided the data summarized herein. Notably absent were reports from Central and South America, Africa, Eastern Europe, Russia and former republics of the Soviet Union, the Middle East (other than Israel), Greenland, and Iceland. Most presenters attempted to gather data from across their regions. Completeness of reports thus varied, depending on the sophistication of the available data collection agencies. Notwithstanding these limitations and omissions, the commonalities and differences revealed in those reports were enlightening and provide an opportunity for fruitful study.

Methods and materials

Reports were heard from New Zealand [2], Canada [3], Asia (Japan) [4], Australia [5], and Europe (France) [6]. Domains responsible for multiple countries varied in data quality. Each reporter made a sincere effort to identify the spectrum of the quality of the data, as well as the opportunities for regional progress. The European and Asian countries solicited for information are identified in Boxes 1 and 2, respectively.

* Department of Orthopedic Surgery, Temple University School of Medicine, 3401 North Broad Street, 6th Floor, Philadelphia, PA 19140.
E-mail address: bertieweiss@hotmail.com

Presenters were given latitude from a guideline PowerPoint file [7] of suggested data. Where available, correlations with financial burdens of the care itself (as opposed to financial burdens on the patients for their lives in general) were identified.

Solicited data points are identified in Box 3.

Results

Incidence rates and demographic patterns varied, largely because of regional social differences as well as differences in data quality or even presence of data collection mechanisms. For example, while Japan had a spinal cord injury registry, none existed for Korea, China, or Pakistan. This made meaningful comparisons of incidences, age distributions, and other factors difficult. Despite these challenges, the disparities observed offered insight into opportunities for a rational approach to assisting underserved regions with sensible mechanisms for lessening the societal and individual burdens associated with tetraplegia.

In the United States, approximately 32 new spinal cord injuries per million people are reported per year. Because of underreporting, the actual number of injuries is likely higher [8,9]. While roughly comparable to the reported Canadian incidence rate, the United States incidence is nearly four times the French experience of only 8 new spinal cord injuries per million population, which, in turn, was similar to the New Zealand experience of 10 per million. Hong Kong's reported incidence of only 1.5 new cases per million reflects the incidence specifically of cervical

0749-0712/08/$ - see front matter © 2008 Elsevier Inc. All rights reserved.
doi:10.1016/j.hcl.2008.01.004

Box 1. European data sources

Austria
Denmark
England
Finland
France
Germany
Greece
Hungary
Italy
Netherlands
Norway
Scotland
Spain
Sweden
Switzerland
Five other (unidentified) European
    countries

Box 3. Solicited data points

Presence of a formal spinal cord injury
    registry
Incidence of spinal cord injuries
Etiology of spinal cord injuries
Demographic distribution of spinal cord
    injuries
Complications of disease and care
Bearer of cost of care (with general fiscal
    environment of health care)
Mechanism of referral to a hand care
    program
Options in nonsurgical management
Techniques and outcomes for surgery
    to restore elbow extension
Techniques and outcomes for surgery to
    restore pinch and grasp
Techniques and outcomes for surgery
    to intrinsic function
Techniques and outcomes for surgery to
    benefit incomplete lesions
Commonly used outcomes measures
Timing for reconstructive upper limb
    surgery postinjury
Age restrictions for reconstructive
    surgery
Common comorbidities

spinal cord injury, since the University of Hong Kong reported a general spinal cord injury incidence of nearly 65 per million population. In the United States, the best data source is the National Spinal Cord Injury Database, which admits it captures all its data from only an estimated 13% of new spinal cord injury cases. Clearly, the data are flawed globally, and reliable estimates of the true incidence regionally simply do not exist.

The United States experience suggests a 3:1 or 4:1 ratio of males to females, with an average age of 28.7 years. Both the median age at injury and the average age of the United States population are increasing, but there is a disparate increase in the percentage of new patients over 60 years of age [8,9].

Reported etiologies were similar, but the differences revealing. Acts of violence, primarily

gunshot wounds, were the third leading cause of spinal cord injury in the United States (13%–25%), and recreational sports were fourth. In France, only 3% of spinal cord injuries were the results of gunshots. Both the United States and Canada identified motor vehicle accidents as the leading cause, while the Australians were more specific in noting that 60% of their injuries resulted from motorcycle accidents. Only the Canadians identified infection on their list.

Financial considerations received less attention than deserved, since this may be where political efforts could result in widely improved opportunities for easing the total burdens borne by these patients. Most Asian countries had no government funding for care, while Canadians and New Zealanders benefited from national insurance. In the United States, those with private insurance were so covered, and those without either exhausted personal funds until eligible for state assistance or qualified for such assistance immediately. When automotive liability insurance was involved, it bore part or the entire burden. That

Box 2. Asian data sources

China
Japan
India
Indonesia
Korea
Pakistan
Malaysia
Singapore
Taiwan
Thailand

burden was substantial, costing between $480,000 and $750,000 the year after injury, and between $55,000 and $133,000 each subsequent year in the United States [8,9].

Lack of referral to a hand program was acknowledged as an impediment to opportunity, identified nearly universally, except in New Zealand, where all upper extremity reconstructions for spinal cord injuries are performed in one center, and all spinal cord injury care is delivered in one of two centers in the country. Through that mechanism, capture of eligible patients for evaluation and education regarding the opportunities available is virtually 100%. In contrast, most Asian countries had few services to offer. Those patients fortunate enough to receive treatment involving a surgeon or occupational therapist aware of reconstructive opportunities would be advised and referred for evaluation. Often, none were involved, and patients who might otherwise benefit were denied those opportunities for the improved independence such procedures offer. Surgeons, physiatrists, and occupational therapists in the United States had varied perceptions of the benefits of upper limb reconstruction. Although all three groups felt that these procedures were of value to their patients, physiatrists rated their perceptions of the benefits lower than surgeons did [10,11].

Agreement was complete that challenges in getting patients to suitable practitioners for evaluation and implementation of upper limb reconstruction were multifactorial and not based on a lack of outcomes data to support the utility of these procedures. Common observations (but without data) also included the tendency for patients to loose interest in reentering the health care system for limb reconstruction once they had "graduated" from the intensive involvement of their first year following injury.

Orthotics were globally used, but reports indicated that use was diminishing in all regions. Most regions supported their use for contracture prevention, and some (Canadians) still recommended tenodesis splints for functional activities. The experience with functional electrical stimulation was mixed, with several speakers expressing reservation about again trying these devices because of poor industry support in the past following implantation, and patient disinterest in the devices after long periods of use and training (France).

Each speaker addressed patterns of preference for surgical reconstructions in three typical functional deficits in the tetraplegic upper limb: elbow extension; grasp, release and pinch; and intrinsic balance. Differences identified were largely based on surgeons' preferences, rather than geography. However, because some regions, such as New Zealand [2], were represented by single centers for reconstruction, their preferences were identical with those of the surgeons operating at their facility. For these reasons, regional differences will not be identified in this section but, rather, generalizations concerning those differences.

Grasp, release, and pinch reconstruction comments indicated common themes, with individual differences based on idiosyncrasies of patients [2–6]. Surgeons differed in their perspectives on the application of the routine use of extensor tenodeses and, when routinely recommending extensor tenodesis, with the use of single- or two-stage reconstructions (for grasp and for release). No other major perspective differences were identified.

For elbow extension transfers, some strongly preferred the biceps to triceps transfer, while others used the deltoid (posterior one half) to triceps transfer [2–6]. Of those preferring the deltoid to the biceps, objections to the latter were based on observed subsequent weakness in elbow flexion and inconsistent restoration of elbow extension strength. Those preferring to use the biceps rather than the deltoid cited more predictable grade 3 or 4 elbow extension and inconsequential loss of elbow flexion strength. Differences were also expressed for the augmentation material used for the deltoid to triceps transfer, including a Dacron weave (Australia [5]) and hamstring grafts (two) (New Zealand [2]). Others described their technique as "standard" (We used a fascial flap from olecranon periosteum continuous with a strip of the central one third of the triceps tendon, reflected proximally).

Incomplete lesions were identified as increasing in frequency, both in terms of absolute numbers of injuries and as a percentage of all spinal cord injuries. It was theorized, without data, that this might be related to an increased awareness of the injuries, as well as an increased opportunity to provide treatment for their impairments to improve the quality of lives. The Japanese [4] noted that most incomplete patients refused surgery. The Australians [5] felt that improvement in neurologic function during the first 12 months postinjury was a contraindication to intervention in patients with incomplete lesions.

Despite requests to consider outcomes measures in the regional perspectives talks, the only speakers to do so were from Japan [4] and Australia [5]. In Japan, the Jebsen tests were preferred, while the Australians relied on muscle strength testing and "patient satisfaction." This reflects the propensity of surgeons to pay little attention to these important tools (see the article by Chung elsewhere in this issue) and reinforces the need for surgeons to work closely with therapists to objectively assess the results of their efforts. Outside the domain of this article, but addressed at the meeting, was an entire precourse session on outcomes. Please see the article by Chung elsewhere in this issue.

Despite previous interest in promoting early intervention for upper limb reconstruction following spinal cord injury, the earliest offer for timing of surgery postinjury came from the French [6], who advised surgery "during the early part of the rehabilitation program," noting that "secondary surgery," defined as surgery after completion of rehabilitation program, was often met with resistance of patients to reenter the health care system. Otherwise, most regions recommended surgery at approximately 1 year postinjury. No one would state an upper limit to age for offering upper limb reconstruction in tetraplegia. To the contrary, as general care improves for tetraplegics, upper limits for reconstruction have disappeared. However, as older patients enjoy the benefits of reconstruction, and as reconstructed patients age, new consequences have appeared, which will need to be addressed. Specifically, the French [6] have seen problems with shoulders in general, and rotator cuffs in particular, in postreconstructed patients.

Finally, the existence of comorbidities drew little comment, suggesting that no one had identified an at-risk population beyond the demographic patterns discussed previously.

Summary

This forum provided an opportunity for exploration of individual and regional differences in surgeons' preferences in tetraplegic upper limb reconstruction, with the goal of determining the best options for these patients. Studies based on outcomes and measured by standardized outcomes testing tools may help direct true differences in treatment offerings.

Improvements are needed in data collection systems, financing of and access to care, especially in underserved regions, and better use of outcomes assessment tools.

References

[1] International Meeting on the Upper Limb in Tetraplegia (video archive). Available at: http://mcjconsulting.com/meeting/2007/tetraplegia/. Accessed March 11, 2008.

[2] Rothwell A. Contemporary trends in the management of upper limb in tetraplegia, New Zealand perspective. Presented at the International Meeting on Upper Limb in Tetraplegia. Philadelphia, September 17–20, 2007.

[3] Kalsi-Ryan S. Contemporary trends in the management of upper limb in tetraplegia, Canadian perspective. Presented at the International Meeting on Upper Limb in Tetraplegia. Philadelphia, September 17–20, 2007.

[4] WY Ip J. Contemporary trends in the management of upper limb in tetraplegia, Asian perspective. Presented at the International Meeting on Upper Limb in Tetraplegia. Philadelphia, September 17–20, 2007.

[5] Flood S. Contemporary trends in the management of upper limb in tetraplegia, Australian perspective. Presented at the International Meeting on Upper Limb in Tetraplegia. Philadelphia, September 17–20, 2007.

[6] Leclercq C. Contemporary trends in the management of upper limb in tetraplegia, European perspective. Presented at the International Meeting on Upper Limb in Tetraplegia. Philadelphia, September 17–20, 2007.

[7] Mulcahey MJ. Contemporary trends in the management of upper limb in tetraplegia: a sample PowerPoint presentation. Presented at the International Meeting on Upper Limb in Tetraplegia. Philadelphia, September 17–20, 2007.

[8] National Spinal Cord Injury Statistical Center. 2006 fact sheet. Available at: http://www.spinalcord.uab.edu/show.asp?durki=21446. Accessed March 11, 2008.

[9] National Spinal Cord Injury Resource Center. Available at: http://www.sci-info-pages.com/factsheets.html#Factsheet%20#2. Accessed March 11, 2008.

[10] Curtin CM, Hayward RA, Kim M, et al. Physician perceptions of upper extremity reconstruction of the person with tetraplegia. J Hand Surg [Am] 2005;30(1):87–93.

[11] Friden J, Gohritz A, Ejeskar A. Upper limb surgery in tetraplegic patients over 60 years—You are never too old to improve. Presentation at the International Meeting on Upper Limb in Tetraplegia. Philadelphia, September 17–20, 2007.

Measurement Issues Related to Upper Limb Interventions in Persons Who Have Tetraplegia

Jennifer A. Dunn, Dip PT, MPhil[a], K. Anne Sinnott, Dip PT, MPhty[b,c,*],
Anne M. Bryden, OTR/L[d],
Sandra J. Connolly, BHScOT, OT Reg (Ont)[e],
Alastair G. Rothwell, ONZM, MB, ChM, FRACS[b,c]

[a]*Physiotherapy Department, Burwood Spinal Unit, Private Bag 4708, Christchurch, New Zealand*
[b]*Burwood Spinal Unit, Private Bag 4708, Christchurch, New Zealand*
[c]*Department of Orthopaedic Surgery and Musculoskeletal Medicine, University of Otago,*
Christchurch School of Medicine and Health Sciences, P.O. Box 4710, Christchurch, New Zealand
[d]*The Cleveland Functional Electrical Stimulation Center, MetroHealth Medical Center,*
2500 MetroHealth Drive H601, Cleveland, OH 44109-1998, USA
[e]*St. Joseph's Health Care, Parkwood Hospital, 801 Commissioner's Road East, London, Ontario, Canada N6C 5J1*

As research and technology advance, more innovative treatments for restoring upper extremity function have been developed, resulting in more options for improving hand function and quality of life [1]. The hierarchy for restoration of function starts with maximizing ability based on the person's voluntary function, then augmenting function by implementing technology or advanced innovative interventions. The benefits of innovative interventions of the upper limb specifically for tetraplegia have become well established following the pioneering surgery of Moberg [2], Freehafer [3], Zancolli [4], and Lamb and Chan [5], and the longer-term results of these interventions have been described [6]. A systematic review of the reconstructive surgical interventions for persons with tetraplegia has recently been published [7].

There is increasing recognition of the need to measure health outcomes for clinical, academic, and financial reasons. It is essential to be able to measure outcomes accurately to determine how effective our interventions are. Equally important is the understanding of how rehabilitation works when it is effective. A comprehensive approach to evidence-based rehabilitation will evolve from measuring outcomes, demonstrating how effective our treatment interventions are, and improving our understanding of how the process of rehabilitation relates to effective outcomes. Furthermore, it is important that the consumers of rehabilitation are involved in determining what outcomes are most important.

A theoretic basis for measurement of outcomes exists. The World Health Organization (WHO) International Classification of Function, Disability and Health (ICF) [8] was developed to provide a better understanding of the consequences of disabling conditions. It divides the consequences of injury or illness into various domains at two distinctive levels, which (the authors believe) provides a framework on which to base outcome measurement (Fig. 1). The development of the ICF Core Set for SCI Project is based on the premise that sound measurement of the consequences of spinal cord injury (SCI) is required at these distinctive levels. Biering-Sorensen and colleagues [9] emphasize that an important basis for the optimum acute and long-term management of SCI is an in-depth understanding, systematic consideration, and

* Corresponding author. Rehabilitation Teaching and Research Unit, University of Otago, PO Box 7343, Wellington South, New Zealand.

E-mail address: anne.sinnott@otago.ac.nz
(K.A. Sinnott).

0749-0712/08/$ - see front matter © 2008 Elsevier Inc. All rights reserved.
doi:10.1016/j.hcl.2008.01.005

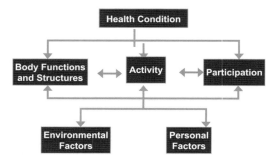

Fig. 1. International Classification of Functioning, Disability and Health (ICF) (WHO 2001). (*From* World Health Organisation. International classification of functioning, disability and health. Geneva (Switzerland): World Health Organisation; 2002; with permission.)

sound measurement of the consequences of living with this chronic disabling condition. This includes the consumer or patient perspective.

The ICF offers some practical assistance when faced with the choice of measurement tools available and the objectives of measuring. The focus and scope of measurement are sometimes used interchangeably but it is less confusing and more accurate to define them in the following way. *Focus* is about what the measure is directed to and getting information about. For example, is the *focal point* body structure or function, activity or participation, or something else? In contrast, the *scope* of the measure means how broad or extensive the measure might be. For example, the focal point is activities but the scope would be hand-based activities of daily living (ADL) for people with tetraplegia after tendon transfer surgery. The mathematical properties of the measure is referred to as the level. These levels include nominal, ordinal, interval, and ratio data, and the distinct characteristics that differentiate these different levels. The main result is that the level determines how scores or numbers used in the measure can be interpreted.

Persons with tetraplegia at the level of C5, C6, or C7 have little active movement below the elbow, which limits not only arm and hand movement but also their ability to perform ADL, such as eating, grooming, and communication. Generally, on discharge from a rehabilitation program, persons with C5 tetraplegia are able to feed themselves with assistive devices, but remain dependent for transferring into and out of a wheelchair, for bladder and bowel care, and will usually use a power wheelchair for community mobility. Persons with C6 and C7 tetraplegia, having normal wrist

extension power, use a passive tenodesis grip, which makes weak grasp and gravity release possible. The passive tenodesis grasp occurs because the tendons of the main finger flexors and extensor pass over the wrist and therefore motion of the wrist puts one or other group of tendons under tension. Thus, when a C6 or C7 person with tetraplegia extends his or her wrist, the fingers and thumb automatically flex, allowing for a weak lateral and gross grip pattern. Conversely gravity-assisted wrist flexion tightens the finger and thumb extensors, enabling grasp release. Because of this grasp pattern, persons with C6 or C7 tetraplegia are generally able to dress the upper half of their body, may be able to transfer themselves on and off a wheelchair, are more efficient in using a manual wheelchair, but still require assistance with bowel care and assistance with appliances for bladder drainage.

Nonsurgical restoration of hand function in tetraplegia usually encompasses the use of adaptive devices, positioning, and compensatory movements. Most people with tetraplegia strive to look and act "normal" when using their hands. Therefore, dependence on bulky feeding splints, adapted equipment, and physical assistance in performing personal tasks encourages many tetraplegic persons to consider any one of a variety of surgical interventions.

Individuals with tetraplegia receive conservative treatment at various stages of their rehabilitation to maximize upper extremity function [10]. More innovative approaches for restoring upper extremity function have been tried and the process for choosing such interventions has been documented [11], but is beyond the scope of this article.

This complex process depends on many factors, such as how satisfied the individual is with his or her residual function, the quality of conservative treatment received, whether he or she has been exposed to surgical procedures to restore function, the individual's overall health status, and the person's ability to tolerate surgery and the rehabilitation process that follows [6].

Measurement of outcomes to determine the consequences of upper limb interventions for persons with tetraplegia is necessary to increase our understanding about the nature and natural history of tetraplegia [1]. Measurements assist in evaluating interventions and the efficiency of rehabilitation programs to restore hand function. Merely choosing a popular measure of the day may mean that important questions are overlooked, such as "Why measure?" and "What shall we measure?" [12]. That is, before choosing what should be measured, one needs to be clear about the purpose of the measurement [12]. In evaluating interventions, we agree that one should measure those factors likely to be affected by the intervention, those that might be affected, and those factors quite unlikely to be affected. It is obvious that such a comprehensive approach is not always feasible and those outcomes concerned with effectiveness may need priority over those reflecting efficiency [12].

Assessment and measurement are complex processes [12,13]. They require the integration of information from a variety of sources and rely on clinical skills for interpretation. Assessment can indeed be performed without standardized measures, which is an appropriate course of action at times. It is important to know when and when not to use standardized measures. It is equally important to recognize the limits of assessment without measurement and measurement without assessment. To interpret information from measures requires an understanding of measurement itself and the context of its use. The use of standardized outcome measures allows surgeons, physicians, therapists, and scientists involved in the surgery and rehabilitation of the upper limb in tetraplegia to make a clear distinction between the process of assessment (requiring interpretation) and that of measurement (the quantification of an observation against a standard) to determine the consequences of the reconstructive upper limb interventions.

In the first instance, the most effective methodology for finding out how much function is to make measurements before intervention and to repeat the same measures following intervention. In practice, this methodology is not that simple. Although often viewed as synonymous, and frequently used interchangeably, outcome measures are not the same thing as diagnostic measures, which in turn are not the same thing as prognostic measures. It is crucial that the distinctions are made and understood. Measurements are taken for a number of reasons: to diagnose a condition, to measure the severity or extent of a feature present in an individual, to make a prognosis about a condition, to evaluate change over time, to measure the consequences of an intervention, and to evaluate effectiveness of a program. A single measure is not necessarily capable of achieving more than one purpose. The properties of predictive and diagnostic measures are different from those of evaluative or outcome measures. When talking

about "outcome measurement," not only do we need to know whether we are talking about prognosis, diagnosis, or outcomes, we also need to clearly state the level being measured so that the interpretation of measures will be more meaningful [12,13].

These complexities are ever present when we consider the measurement of the outcomes of upper limb interventions for persons with tetraplegia. The decision to use more innovative approaches to restore upper extremity function carries a responsibility to employ an open and comprehensive assessment methodology capable of capturing both anticipated and unforeseen consequences for the individual. The sudden transition from relative good health and function to a state of impairment and dysfunction, including the loss of upper limb function, is devastating to the individual.

The primary purpose of this article is to explore six fundamental issues that impact both the processes of measurement and the interpretation of the data from standardized outcome measurements. The subsequent discussion focuses on how best we might use the ICF to harness our combined energies more efficiently and holistically in terms of improved functioning and well-being for this consumer group.

Measurement issues

Comprehensive physiologic evaluation

First, despite the evolution and development of specific classification schemes, such as the American Spinal Injury Association (ASIA) scoring system, the International Standards for Neurologic and Functional Classification of SCI [14], and the International Classification for Surgery of the Hand [15], important pieces are still missing from the comprehensive physiologic evaluation necessary to determine the best and most appropriate options for restoring upper extremity function. Specifically, measures of denervation and spasticity remain lacking [16]. The innervation status of the paralyzed muscles is important. The type of paralysis determines what methods of intervention for improving upper extremity function will be most effective, such as tendon transfers versus functional electrical stimulation. Additionally, the presence of lower motor neuron damage can place an individual at risk for contracture development in the antagonist voluntary muscle. It is important to identify this risk early after the injury so that preventative therapies may be employed or the decision to intervene surgically can be made. In addition, autonomic function should be adequately assessed and classified. It is beyond the scope of this article to explore this in depth, but it appears that autonomic functions influence hand function and performance.

Hand ability versus activities-of-daily-living performance

Second, activity performance must be divided into two categories when considering upper extremity function after tetraplegia: hand ability and ADL performance. The category of hand ability would include tests designed to look at the person's ability to manipulate and hold or move different objects. By comparison, the category of ADL performance includes tests that measure the person's ability to use his or her hand functionally to perform daily tasks. It is important be clear about such distinctions and to evaluate function in both categories. The ICF makes a clear distinction between capacity and performance [8], facilitating the assessment of what activities people actually can do with their hands separate from what activities they perform with their hands in their home environment.

Many of the existing tests of hand and ADL function are not appropriate for measuring the changes in function in people with tetraplegia [17]. The necessary criteria for choosing an appropriate test have been stated [1] and include (1) activities appropriate for tetraplegic individuals representing their ability to perform actual ADLs requiring hand function, (2) insensitivity to learning, (3) standardized administration, (4) an unambiguous scale that does not combine too many aspects of function (ie, level of independence and time for completion scored concurrently), (5) multiple trials to help ensure reliability, and (6) sensitivity to changes provided by treatment or intervention to restore upper extremity function. While many tests have been used with people with SCI [18–24], there is still a great need to increase their overall sensitivity to detect small but meaningful changes in this population, as well as to improve the specificity in the scoring of these changes.

Recognition of contextual factors

Third, environmental and personal factors, such as gender, race, age, social background, past life events, character style, or other health conditions that are not part of the health condition or health state, have an impact on the individual's response to the rehabilitation demands of any upper limb interventions. Measurement of these contextual factors is not straightforward, but such measurement may exhibit the greatest difference perceived as significant by the individual [25]. For example, in some cultures it is the family's responsibility to take care of the person who is injured, possibly limiting the person's ability to be more independent.

Timed testing

Next, many of the existing tests rely on timed testing of tasks to determine changes in function following an upper limb intervention. However, the fundamental issue here is that it is not the time taken to perform the task that is of key concern to the individual, but the ability to perform the task and, further, the ability to perform the task consistently.

For the individual with tetraplegia, the decision to perform ADL does not hinge on the time taken but rather the safety, independence, and performance consistency of the task. Therefore when addressing changes in hand function, tests that measure ability to perform suitable tasks and consistency in this performance give a better understanding of tetraplegic hand function than those that rely on timed testing. The Capabilities of the Upper Extremity [26] and the Van Lieshout Test Short Form [27,28] are two such tests. Additionally, the Grasp Release Test developed by Woulle and colleagues [24] measures both completions and failures in functionally specific tasks to measure tetraplegic hand ability within a set time period, rather than timing the task completion.

Timing of measurement

In addition, the consideration of time is important in a temporal sense. As persons with SCI survive longer, problems arise because of aging of various anatomic and physiologic systems superimposed on a pre-existing disability. This has to be a major consideration with upper limb reconstructive interventions and the interventions over time from the perspective of all parties. Adequate measurement is required to demonstrate that interventions are both desired and effective over the lifetime of the individual. How persons with tetraplegia benefit from a particular intervention may not always be obvious, but will be even less obvious if not measured or only measured from one perspective over time.

For example, with the use of a framework, such as the ICF, the focus of interest changes with time from the health condition to the changes in activity or level of participation, and from the person to his or her environment [25,29].

Ownership of the outcomes of interest

Finally, there is a fundamental requirement to collaborate with the person living with the health condition to gain insights into his or her individual perspective. This is not to suggest in this context that the individual is an expert on upper limb interventions for tetraplegia. However, that person is the expert on his or her life with tetraplegia in his or her environmental and personal context [25]. This may sound simplistic, but as health professionals we are ethically bound to truly explore that context.

Discussion

The ICF is essentially a classification system— a taxonomy for deciding what to measure, in relation to functioning, rather than how to measure. The aim of the ICF is to provide a unified and standard language and framework for the description of health and health-related outcomes. It provides a useful framework for organizing our knowledge, planning, and case formulation in the clinical setting, as well as a basis for interpreting measurement. For example, following a reconstructive forearm tendon transfer procedure, the focus of care may indeed be more heavily weighted in the domain of body functions and structures, both subjectively and objectively, during the initial postoperative phase.

There may be a subtle shift toward real-life participation and the possibility of a change in life roles as the person gains small but meaningful hand function. Obviously, it is crucial that each domain receives some attention during every phase following upper limb interventions with consistent attention to measuring the subtle changes over time at the individual level. A measure at the body structures and body functions level may be best interpreted in light of an activity measure used to determine the extent of real-life participation. The ICF reinforces the notion that rehabilitation is not just about disablement or independence, but also offers a way of thinking about the consequences of disabling conditions that means rehabilitation professionals become aware of the role of functional limitations (and natural recovery) as well as the contextual factors that are so important for all humans.

In the first instance, the health condition is usually the cause of impairments to body structures and body functions, which lead to activity limitations, which lead to the participation restrictions. While perhaps at risk of being too simplistic, consideration of measurement at these specific levels can be useful. Although the parameters are intertwined, each is unique and can contribute to the overall interpretation of the level of disablement of an individual. It is also well established that the relationship between these parameters is not linear. The magnitude of the level of restrictions in participation results not only from the interaction of the impairments to body structures and body functions and limitations in activity, but also from the person's physical environment, social and economic setting, and the resources available.

Interestingly, it was suggested at the 7th International Tetraplegia and Upper Limb Surgery meeting (Bologna, Italy, 2001) that a consensus on outcome measurement be sought based on the WHO framework. At the time, the version in use was the International Classification of Impairment Disability and Handicap (ICIDH-2) [30]. While this seemed logical and reasonable, international agreement did not occur.

When one speaks of "outcome measurement" it is simply that—the measurement of the consequences for the individual person. This is a simple notion, yet one that frequently eludes clinicians as we drown in the morass of choices. With use of the ICF taxonomy, we ought to be well placed to recognize the strengths and weaknesses within the concepts of assessment and measurement and to agree on how to use standardized outcome measures to determine, at the very least, the consequences over time of a person's level of impairment to body structures and functions, and to what extent that level of impairment limits activities and restricts participation [25,29].

The lack of agreed methods for interpretation of measurement tools is impeding progress. One way to improve the sharing of information is to make systematic, detailed observations using psychometrically sound measures within an agreed framework, thereby replacing ambiguity and confusion with greater accuracy and discrimination. Agreement of a common language is vital. Without some sort of framework or theoretic basis, any description of outcome is likely to be inadequate. Whether we like it or not, all rehabilitation ought to be undertaken with a theory in mind and for now the ICF appears to be the agreed international theoretic construct [31]. It is reassuring to see that the desire for such international agreement was endorsed at the recent 9th International Tetraplegia and Upper Limb Surgery scientific meeting in Philadelphia.

Further to the ICF perspective, we wish to make four points of interest relating to the measurement of outcomes for this consumer group. First, it has become more obvious over time that more careful consideration of a participant's perspective of "successful outcome" involves some level of reflection on the part of the individual of preinjury lifestyle, dreams, aspirations, and goals—preinjury motivators and inherent skills. It seems reasonable that for any of us, the perspective of "successful outcome" might be influenced by our past experience and successes or failures that make up such experiences. One such consideration is the suggestion that what may have worked for the individual in terms of coping mechanisms preinjury is likely to be the best place to start postinjury [32].

A second consideration is the actual learning process of motor skill acquisition. In the New Zealand study [6,29], patients reported that they learned to "move" their reconstructed hands during postoperative rehabilitation following bilateral simultaneous forearm tendon transfer surgery, but learned to "use" their reconstructed hands once home in their own environment doing "their own thing through trial and error" [29]. Further, it was reported that this process continued for up to 3 to 5 years postsurgery. Not only does this raise interest in terms of the environmental influences, it emphasizes the significance of individual goal-directed learning, the impact of time, and learning through the personal experience of performing [33].

The notion of participation in terms of motor skill acquisition is the third consideration. While acknowledging the difficulties involved, it seems reasonable to explore this domain in relation to the barriers and facilitators to the learning process. It has been acknowledged that there are various learning styles in childhood that are more or less successful for each of us. We suggest that, in terms of learning following SCI, what previously worked for an individual preinjury may be relevant postinjury [32,33].

Yet, there is little consideration, if any, of preinjury experiences, skills, or successful motor skill acquisition for these persons with tetraplegia either contemplating or recovering from surgery. For example, in practice, it appears to be the combination of key pinch and hook grips and the synergic actions of the innervated muscles, transposed tendons, stabilized joints, and reconstructed thumb position that provides the functional advantage from forearm tendon transfer surgery [6]. The functional gains include a variety of previously unachievable fine arm-hand activities with considerable variation in participation, a natural consequence for those who choose to maximize the opportunity. In terms of motor skill acquisition, the transposing of tendons that then demands complex synergic muscle activity places extraordinary demands on the patient during postoperative rehabilitation. Interestingly, in the rehabilitation literature about upper limb reconstructive interventions, little mention is made of movement coordination, let alone personal motivation and individual goal-directed learning associated with task completion.

Finally, we mention research methodology. At the 8th International Upper Limb Surgery and Tetraplegia scientific meeting (Christchurch, New Zealand, 2004), only one of a small number of research groups was using qualitative research methods as a method of enquiry. While this move to incorporate qualitative methodology in New Zealand is relatively recent, the single case study has been undertaken as a pilot study using Grounded Theory methods and interpreted using the ICF [33]. We explored the concept of "life impact" in terms of participation, learning experiences, and hand motor skills.

In full knowledge of the limitation of this single case design, we use it merely as an example to demonstrate the practical use of the ICF as the basis of interpretation of measurements. First, within the domain of "body structures and functions" the participant emphasized enhancement in relation to manual dexterity (hand grip and strength) and mobility. Second, in the domain of activity, facilitation was identified with regard to manual performance (including lifting and grasping objects), personal care, and communication (specifically handwriting). Third, within "participation," improvements were identified in relation to engagement in employment, recreation, and social interaction. Next, in the context of "environmental factors," benefits were noted in regard to improved ability to gain access to different environments and to use advances in technology (including cell phones, swipe cards, wheelchairs, and vehicle modifications). Finally, with regard to "personal factors," the participant identified key impacts related to improved confidence, self-image, and self-esteem.

Taking this further, we suggest that, in a sense, the upper limb surgical intervention appeared to unlock the potential to effectively use additional environmental improvements that occurred over time, and to reassert the determination and inherent abilities evident before SCI. In this regard, while the technological advances previously described, together with improved access to buildings and transport and greater social acceptance of disability over time were regarded as highly significant facilitators, the upper limb surgical intervention was identified as the single most important life-changing event.

This notion is aptly portrayed by the following verbatim quote from an enthusiastic consumer: "I had the functional use of my hands back. For someone with previously so little, this was so much."

Recommendations

First, it was agreed at the 9th International Upper Limb Surgery and Tetraplegia scientific meeting (Philadelphia, September 2007) that the ICF be adopted to theoretically underpin outcomes research by this group. Second, following the recommendation made in Christchurch in 2004, it was agreed to include the Canadian Occupational Performance Measure [34] as a common measure. The final recommendation was that an international collaborative effort be made to undertake a prospective cohort study to allow for a greater sample size and therefore study power, but also to lift the level of study design further up the accepted hierarchy. Work is now underway to design a suitably acceptable study protocol using a battery of outcome measures. This study needs outcome measures to be validated in a variety of languages to enable international collaboration. The systematic review undertaken by Connolly and colleagues [7] will be a starting point.

Summary

While the ICF provides the framework for the measurement and interpretation of outcomes, attention should still be directed toward choosing appropriate outcome measures for detecting the often subtle, yet significant functional gains.

International agreement is required. The most important contribution of the ICF is the focus on all aspects of human function from the basics of movement to participation in life in a personally meaningful way by considering all domains throughout the entire rehabilitation process.

References

[1] Bryden AM, Sinnott KA, Mulcahey MJ. Innovative strategies for improving upper extremity function in persons with tetraplegia and considerations in measuring functional outcomes. Topics in Spinal Cord Injury Rehabilitation 2005;10(4):75–93.

[2] Moberg E. Surgical rehabilitation of the upper limb in tetraplegia. Paraplegia 1990;74B(6):873–9.

[3] Freehafer AA. Tendon transfers in patients with cervical spinal cord injury. J Hand Surg [Am] 1991; 16:804–9.

[4] Zancolli EA. Surgery for the quadriplegic hand with active, strong wrist extension preserved. Clin Orthop Relat Res 1975;112:101–13.

[5] Lamb DW, Chan KM. Surgical reconstruction of the upper limb in traumatic tetraplegia. J Bone Joint Surg Br 1983;65:291–8.

[6] Rothwell AG, Sinnott KA, Mohammed KD, et al. Upper limb surgery for tetraplegia: a 10-year re-review of hand function. J Hand Surg [Am] 2003; 28:489–97.

[7] Connolly SJ, Aubut JL, Teasell R, et al. Enhancing upper extremity function with reconstructive surgery in persons with tetraplegia: a review of the literature. Topics in Spinal Cord Injury Rehabilitation 2007; 13(1):58–80.

[8] World Health Organisation. International classification of functioning, disability and health. Geneva (Switzerland): World Health Organisation; 2002.

[9] Biering-Sorensen F, Scheuringer M, Baumberger M, et al. Developing core sets for persons with spinal cord injuries based on the International Classification of Functioning, Disability and Health as a way to specify functioning. Spinal Cord 2006; 44(9):541–6.

[10] Curtin M. Development of a tetraplegic hand assessment and splinting protocol. Paraplegia 1994; 32:159–69.

[11] Snoek GJ, Ijzerman MJ, Hermens HJ, et al. Survey of the needs of patients with spinal cord injury: impact and priority for improvement in hand function in tetraplegics. Spinal Cord 2004;42(9):526–32.

[12] Wade D. Measurement in neurological rehabilitation. Oxford (UK): Oxford University Press; 1992.

[13] Whiteneck GG. Measuring what matters: key rehabilitation outcomes. Arch Phys Med Rehabil 1994; 75:1073–6.

[14] Maynard FM, Bracken MB, Creasy G, et al. International standards for neurological and functional

classification of spinal cord injury. Spinal Cord 1997;35:266–74.

[15] McDowell CL, Moberg E, House JH. The Second International Conference on Surgical Rehabilitation of the Upper Limb in Tetraplegia (Quadriplegia). J Hand Surg [Am] 1986;11A(4):604–8.

[16] Bryden AM, Kilgore KL, Lind BB, et al. Triceps denervation as a predictor of elbow flexion contractures in C5 and C6 tetraplegia. Arch Phys Med Rehabil 2004;85:1880–5.

[17] van Tuijl JH, Janssen-Potten YJ, Seelen HA. Evaluation of upper extremity motor function tests in tetraplegics. Spinal Cord 2002;40(2):51–64.

[18] Klein RM, Bell B. Self-care skills: behavioral measurement with Klein-Bell ADL scale. Arch Phys Med Rehabil 1982;63:335–8.

[19] Catz A, Itzkovich M, Agranov E, et al. SCIM—spinal cord independence measure: a new disability scale for patients with spinal cord lesions. Spinal Cord 1997;35:850–6.

[20] Gresham GE, Labi MLC, Dittmar SS, et al. The Quadriplegia Index of Function (QIF): sensitivity and reliability demonstrated in a study of thirty quadriplegic patients. Paraplegia 1986;24:38–44.

[21] Mahoney FI, Barthel DW. Functional evaluation: the Barthel Index. Md State Med J 1965;14:61–5.

[22] Hamilton BB, Laughlin JA, Fielder RC, et al. Inter-rater reliability of the 7 level functional independence measure (FIM). Scandinavian Journal of Rehabilitation Medicine 1994;26(3):115–9.

[23] Hamilton BB, Granger CV, Sherwin FS, et al. A uniform national data system for medical rehabilitation. In: Fuhrer MJ, editor. Rehabilitation outcomes: analysis and measurement. Baltimore (MD): Paul Brookes Publishing; 1987. p. 133–52.

[24] Woulle K, Van Doren Van CL, Thrope GB, et al. Development of a quantitative hand grasp and release test for patients with tetraplegia using a hand neuroprosthesis. J Hand Surg [Am] 1994;19(A):209–18.

[25] Stucki G, Ewart T, Cieza A. Value and application of the ICF in rehabilitation medicine. Disabil Rehabil 2003;25(11–12):628–34.

[26] Marino RJ, She JA, Stineman MG. The capabilities of upper extremity instrument: reliability and validity of a measure of functional limitation in tetraplegia. Arch Phys Med Rehabil 1998;79:1512–21.

[27] Spooren AI, Janssen-Potten YJ, Post MW, et al. Measuring change in arm hand skilled performance in persons with a cervical spinal cord injury: responsiveness of the Van Lieshout Test. Spinal Cord 2006;44(12):772–9.

[28] Post MW, Van Lieshout G, Seelen HA, et al. Measurement properties of the short version of the Van Lieshout test for arm/hand function of persons with tetraplegia after spinal cord injury. Spinal Cord 2006;44(12):763–71.

[29] Sinnott KA, Dunn JA, Rothwell AG. Use of the ICF conceptual framework to interpret hand function outcomes following tendon transfer surgery for tetraplegia. Spinal Cord 2004;42(7):369–400.

[30] Mulcahey MJ. The overall assessment of the tetraplegic patient. In: The 7th International Conference for Tetraplegia. Bologna (Italy): 2001.

[31] Stucki G, Grimby G. Forward: applying the ICF in medicine. J Rehabil Med 2004;44(Suppl):5–6.

[32] Button C, Davids K, Schollhorn W. Co-ordination profiling of movement systems. In: Davids K, Bennett S, Newell KM, editors. Variability in the movement system: a multi-disiplinary perspective. Champaign (IL): Human Kinetics; 2006. p. 133–52.

[33] Sinnott KA, et al. Life impacts of reconstructive hand surgery in tetraplegia. Topics in Spinal Cord Injury, submitted for publication.

[34] Law M, Baptise S, Carswell A, et al. Canadian occupational performance measure. 3rd edition. Toronto: CAOT Publications; 1998.

ELSEVIER SAUNDERS

Hand Clin 24 (2008) 169–173

HAND
CLINICS

Current Utilization of Reconstructive Upper Limb Surgery in Tetraplegia

Lee Squitieri, BS[a], Kevin C. Chung, MD, MS[b],*

[a]*The University of Michigan Medical School, 1500 E. Medical Center Drive, 2130 Taubman Center, SPC 5340, Ann Arbor, MI 48109, USA*
[b]*Section of Plastic Surgery, Department of Surgery, University of Michigan Health System, 2130 Taubman Center, 1500 E. Medical Center Drive, Ann Arbor, MI 48109-0340, USA*

Upper extremity reconstructive procedures for people with tetraplegia have been described in the literature for more than 60 years. The first surgical technique, presented by Sterling Bunnell in the 1940s, consisted of a series of flexor and extensor tenodesis procedures that provided rudimentary grasp or pinch function to patients able to actively extend and flex their wrists [1–3]. Over time, selected joint fusion procedures were introduced, and in the 1970s, muscle-tendon transfer procedures were proposed as viable reconstructive options. Unfortunately, negative sentiment regarding these procedures quickly arose because of inconsistent success rates, poor patient satisfaction, and the unpredictable spastic nature of many of the transferred muscles [1–7]. The persistence of these pessimistic attitudes over time has generated a negative bias among many caregivers—physiatrists, therapists, and surgeons—regarding current reconstructive techniques. As a result, splinting and external devices are often employed at the exclusion of surgical measures [8–10].

Current classification, evaluation, and treatment

Given the varied presentation of cervical neurologic defects in tetraplegic patients and thus the individualized nature of reconstructive treatment options, surgeons treating this patient population require a precise, comprehensive method for evaluating residual function that enables them to correlate their findings with a practical treatment plan [1,11]. The International Classification for Surgery of the Hand in Tetraplegia (ICSHT) is a tool for evaluating the motor function for each muscle below the elbow and for assessing the thumb and index fingers. This classification is used by all surgeons involved in upper extremity care for tetraplegic patients [12]. Unlike the International Standards for Neurologic Classification of Spinal Cord Injury motor and sensory examinations, which are primarily used by other clinicians to assess residual function, the ICSHT system is specifically designed to assess muscle strength within the context of surgical eligibility and planning [13]. Proper assignment of patients into the appropriate ICSHT subgroup generally determines the goals of reconstructive treatment as well as procedure eligibility [14]. Table 1 lists the treatment goals and suitable procedures for each category of patients as determined by the ICSHT system.

Underutilization of reconstructive procedures

Based on the above surgical classification scheme, leaders in this field have estimated that 60% to 75% of tetraplegic patients are candidates for some type of upper extremity reconstruction [15–18]. A recent study examining the health and treatment priorities among a sample of tetraplegic patients in the United States demonstrated that 42% of tetraplegic patients view upper limb function as their top restoration desire (ie, the function they would want restored first), and 44% of

This article was supported in part by a Mid-career Investigator Award in Patient-Oriented Research (K24 AR053120) from the National Institute of Arthritis and Musculoskeletal and Skin Diseases (Dr. Kevin C. Chung).

* Corresponding author.
E-mail address: kecchung@umich.edu (K.C. Chung).

0749-0712/08/$ - see front matter © 2008 Elsevier Inc. All rights reserved.
doi:10.1016/j.hcl.2008.01.001

hand.theclinics.com

Table 1
ICSHT system

Sensibility[a]	Motor characteristics	Description of function	Treatment goal	Appropriate surgical procedures
0	No muscles below elbow suitable for transfer	Flexion-supination of elbow	Any improvement	Wrist fusion; the Brummer winch operation; functional neuromuscular stimulation
1	Brachioradialis			Strengthening wrist extension[b]
2	Extensor carpi radialis longus	Extension of wrist (weak or strong)	Improved wrist control with or without weak grasp	The Möberg key-grip procedure
3	Extensor carpi radialis brevis[c]	Extension of wrist	Strong wrist extension (if necessary) and grasp	Transfer of the brachioradialis to the flexor pollicis longus, flexor carpi radialis, abductor/extensor pollicis longus, extensor pollicis brevis, or extensor carpi ulnaris
4	Pronator teres	Extension and pronation of wrist	Strong grasp[d]	Transfer of the brachioradialis, one of the extensor carpi radialis muscles, and the pronator teres muscle to power the fingers and thumb
5	Flexor carpi radialis	Flexion of wrist	Opening and closing hand[e]	
6	Finger extensors	Extrinsic extension of fingers, partial or complete		Reconstruction of finger and thumb flexion and intrinsic stabilization
7	Thumb extension	Extrinsic extension of thumb	Intrinsic reconstruction and refined, adaptable function	Tendon transfers to restore or strengthen finger and thumb flexion[f]; dynamic intrinsic substitution procedures to provide digital balance
8	Partial digital flexors	Extrinsic flexion of fingers (weak)		
9	Lacks only intrinsics	Extrinsic flexion of fingers		
X	Exceptions			

A muscle must be at least grade 4 strength to be considered for transfer.
[a] Ocular afferents only or cutaneous sensibility groups.
[b] Requires adequately strong brachioradialis, functional range of passive wrist extension and flexion, shoulder control to assist forearm pronation, and elbow stabilization.
[c] Caution: It is impossible to determine extensor carpi radialis brevis strength without surgical exposure.
[d] May also include stronger group 2 patients.
[e] May also include stronger group 3 patients. Group 3 patients do not have the availability of the pronator teres.
[f] Tendon transfers are only for groups 7 and 8.

Data from Hentz VR, McAdams TR. Restoration of upper extremity function in tetraplegia. In: Hentz VR, editor. Plastic surgery. 2nd edition, vol 8. Philadelphia: Saunders; 2006. p. 507–41; and Hentz VR. Surgical strategy: matching the patient with the procedure. Hand Clin 2002;18:503–18.

surveyed participants reported interest in receiving upper extremity reconstructive surgery [8]. Several case series over the past decade have reviewed the outcomes of these procedures for tetraplegic patients, and the results have been promising [11,19–24]. After reconstruction, patients demonstrated increased pinch force, which improved their ability to eat and write, as well as restored elbow extension, which corresponded with better independent grooming, operation of assisted devices, and the ability to drive automobiles [11,19–24]. Furthermore, in another study surveying tetraplegic patients who received upper extremity surgery, 70% of participants were satisfied with their results and 68% reported improvements in their activities of daily living [25]. These observed patient-rated outcomes are consistent with independently obtained physician estimates of 75% patient satisfaction, suggesting that both patients and their caregivers view surgery to be beneficial and satisfying [8]. However, in spite of these improved outcomes and patient desire for restoration of upper extremity function, a recent study analyzing United States epidemiologic data from 1988 to 2000 found that only 7% of appropriate surgical candidates ultimately receive reconstructive treatment [26]. The results of this study have generated heightened awareness of this problem and precipitated research exploring potential reasons for this profound treatment discrepancy.

One possible explanation for the underutilization of reconstructive surgery may be the lack of clarity in the existing literature about the value of reconstructive procedures. Due to the individualized nature of surgical reconstruction methods for tetraplegic patients, the current available case series are generally small, use inconsistent methods of outcomes reporting, and incorporate a heterogenous collection of different procedures [11,19–24]. The resulting ambiguity makes it difficult for surgeons, physiatrists, and therapists to extrapolate precise risks and benefits of existing procedures, and may cause many clinicians to be wary of recommending reconstruction to patients who cannot afford the potential consequences of surgical risks and further loss of residual function [26].

To date, three studies examining the use of reconstructive surgery among tetraplegics have been published in the literature [8,9,27]. In 2004, Bryden and colleagues [9] surveyed clinicians at 17 of the 18 Model Spinal Cord Injury Centers designated by the U.S. Department of Education's National Institute on Disability Rehabilitation

and Research. The investigators found that 8 of the centers did not offer reconstructive treatment to their patients, with 3 centers citing unavailability of a qualified hand surgeon as a reason, and only 2 of the 17 surveyed physiatrists (12%) had extensive experience (defined as treating > 100 patients) dealing with tetraplegic recipients of reconstructive procedures [9]. Similarly, in a study surveying 455 United States physicians (142 physiatrists and 287 hand surgeons), Curtin and colleagues [27] found that although hand surgeons generally have positive views regarding the effectiveness of upper extremity reconstruction, only 40% of surveyed surgeons reported a desire to perform more of these procedures. Further exploration of this finding revealed that only 42% of hand surgeons felt that their practice was able to accommodate tetraplegic patients [27]. Taken together, the results from both of these studies suggest an acute shortage of surgeons and physiatrists willing or capable of treating these patients, which may contribute to the underutilization of this treatment option.

Other outcomes explored by Curtin and colleagues [27] were differences in caregiver attitudes and predictors of provider performance or referral for upper extremity reconstructive procedures. The results of this study showed that relationships between spinal cord specialists and surgeons have the greatest impact on physician involvement in these procedures. After controlling for all other factors, the investigators found that surgeons who knew spinal cord specialists were 13.1 times more likely to perform upper extremity reconstruction, and physiatrists who maintained relationships with available surgeons were 2.8 times more likely to refer patients for surgery [27]. Thus, the investigators deduced that the greatest barrier to surgical management of tetraplegic patients is the absence of coordinated cross-specialty relationships between surgeons and physiatrists. This conclusion is logical in the context of a shortage in caregiver supply because both surgeons and spinal cord specialists have decreased opportunities to develop close interdisciplinary relationships and also lack sufficient time to comanage surgically treated tetraplegic patients.

In addition, the results of Curtin's study also showed that while both specialties agreed that upper extremity reconstructive procedures were effective, surgeons were significantly more positive than physiatrists regarding treatment outcomes [27]. To determine the impact of negative physician biases toward reconstructive surgery on procedure use, Wagner and colleagues [8] administered an oral survey to a sample of 50 tetraplegic patients and found that patients who learned about reconstructive procedures from physicians were significantly more likely to have a negative first impression of surgery (67% versus 19%, respectively; $P = .004$), less likely to believe that these procedures would improve their independence (60% versus 100%, respectively; $P = .01$), less likely to believe that these procedures would improve their quality of life (53% versus 95%, respectively; $P = .02$), and less likely to believe that the gains were worth the risks of surgery. Furthermore, after controlling for age, gender, and time since injury, the investigators found that learning about reconstructive surgery from someone other than a physician was the only significant positive predictor of a patient wanting surgery (odds ratio: 15.7) [8]. These data attest to the substantial influence that physician counseling has on patient perception, and also identify the presence of a substantial negative bias among physicians toward upper extremity surgery. Ultimately, the investigators concluded that the lack of awareness and negative first impression among tetraplegic patients about upper extremity reconstructive procedures has also contributed to the low use of these treatment options.

Wagner and colleagues [8] also examined the influence of cost and coverage on the utility of reconstructive procedures from the patient perspective. Although 20 out of 50 patients (40%) reported concern about the cost of the surgical procedure, this factor was not found to have a substantial impact on patient desire for reconstruction when analyzed using a logistic regression model. It is revealing to compare these findings with those of Bryden and colleagues [9], who found that the primary reason that treatment centers did not offer upper extremity surgery was a perceived lack of insurance coverage. Together these results show that, in weighing the utility of reconstructive surgery, cost and coverage issues have more impact on caregivers than on tetraplegic patients. Four out of 18 Model Spinal Cord Injury Centers do not offer surgical treatment options, because they assume patients do not have insurance coverage or are unwilling to pay, even though many patients have such coverage or are willing to pay [8,9]. Thus, the lack of clinician and treatment center awareness and education regarding the process of obtaining reimbursement represents another barrier to upper extremity reconstruction surgery for tetraplegic patients.

Inherent weaknesses of the tetraplegic patient population

As economic pressures continue to affect medicine, it will become increasingly important to ensure that vulnerable patient populations continue to have access to appropriate health care. Unlike other disabled patients who suffer from less severe limitations and may be able to live more independently, tetraplegic patients must endure the combined limitations of wheelchair status as well as the inability to use their arms and hands to manipulate devices. Transportation restrictions and problems operating common methods of communication, such as the telephone or computer, make it difficult for these patients to independently obtain information outside of their scheduled physician visits about their medical condition and treatment options. Thus, for tetraplegic patients, the task of obtaining the required approval from physicians and therapists for surgery referral is more cumbersome and complicated than for most other patients. The complex disabilities of tetraplegic patients also impair their ability to organize and influence policy and reimbursement changes regarding their health status. Considering the unique challenges faced by this patient population, it is critical for caregivers to provide adequate access to information and treatment.

Summary

Much of the functional disability associated with tetraplegia results from impaired use of the upper limbs, and 42% of patients who have tetraplegia rated upper extremity function as their top restoration desire [8]. While upper extremity reconstructive surgery has been shown to substantially improve upper limb function and enhance patient independence, recent studies have demonstrated that these procedures are rarely performed and profoundly underutilized [8,9,11,19–27]. As the providers of upper extremity reconstructive surgery, hand surgeons must take a leadership role in promoting greater use of these procedures for tetraplegic patients. Given the complex, multifaceted nature of this dilemma, our recommendations for a future course of action involve both educational and research components.

We believe that constructive collaboration between hand surgery and physiatry societies is the first step toward improved conjoint care for this patient population. In addition, we recommend the development of new and improved outcomes assessment tools specific to the unique needs of tetraplegic patients and the use of these tools in future controlled clinical trials. Through the results of these future trials and systematic reviews, physicians will better understand specific outcomes and complication rates for the various upper extremity reconstructive procedures. Once physicians become more knowledgeable regarding the specific risks and benefits of these procedures, they will be able to accurately counsel tetraplegic patients about surgical options. Finally, efforts should be made to ensure that centers of excellence for upper extremity reconstruction are available to the entire tetraplegic population.

Acknowledgments

The authors appreciate the guidance of Drs. Rod Hentz and Michael Keith in their tireless efforts to help structure the upper extremity reconstructive program at the University of Michigan for people with tetraplegia.

References

[1] Hentz VR, McAdams TR. Restoration of upper extremity function in tetraplegia. In: Hentz VR, editor. Plastic Surgery. 2nd edition, vol 8. Philadelphia: Saunders; 2006. p. 507–41

[2] Bunnell S. Surgery of the hand. Philadelphia: JB Lippincott; 1944.

[3] Bunnell S. Tendon transfer in the hand and forearm. American Academy of Orthopaedic Surgeons Instructional Course Lectures 1949;6:106–12.

[4] Nickel VL, Perry J, Garret AL. Development of useful function in the severely paralyzed hand. J Bone Joint Surg 1963;45:933–52.

[5] Lamb DW, Landry R. The hand in quadriplegia. Hand 1971;3:31–7.

[6] Zancolli E. Structural and dynamic basis of hand surgery. Philadelphia: JB Lippincott; 1968.

[7] Guttmann L. Spinal cord injuries: comprehensive management and research. 2nd edition. Oxford: Blackwell Scientific; 1976.

[8] Wagner JP, Curtin CM, Gater DR, et al. Perceptions of people with tetraplegia regarding surgery to improve upper-extremity function. J Hand Surg [Am] 2007;32A:483–90.

[9] Bryden AM, Wuolle KS, Murray PK, et al. Perceived outcomes and utilization of upper extremity surgical reconstruction in individuals with tetraplegia at model spinal cord injury systems. Spinal Cord 2004;42:169–76.

[10] Snoek GJ, IJzerman MJ, Hermens HJ, et al. Survey of the needs of patients with spinal cord injury: impact and priority for improvement in hand function in tetraplegics. Spinal Cord 2004;42:526–32.

[11] Forner-Cordero I, Mudarra-Garcia J, Forner-Valero JV, et al. The role of upper limb surgery in tetraplegia. Spinal Cord 2003;41:90–6.

[12] McDowell CL, Moberg EA, House JH. The second international conference on surgical rehabilitation of the upper limb in traumatic quadriplegia. J Hand Surg [Am] 1986;11A:604–8.

[13] Mulcahey MJ, Hutchinson D, Kozin S. Assessment of upper limb in tetraplegia: considerations in evaluation and outcomes research. J Rehab Res Dev 2007; 41:91–102.

[14] Hentz VR. Surgical strategy: matching the patient with the procedure. Hand Clin 2002;18:503–18.

[15] Moberg E. Surgical treatment for absent single-hand grip and elbow extension in quadriplegia. Principles and preliminary experience. J Bone Joint Surg 1975; 57A:196–206.

[16] Hentz VR, Brown M, Keoshian LA. Upper limb reconstruction in quadriplegia: functional assessment and proposed treatment modifications. J Hand Surg [Am] 1983;8:119–31.

[17] Nobunaga AI, Go BK, Karunas RB. Recent demographic and injury trends in people served by the model spinal cord injury care systems. Arch Phys Med Rehabil 1999;80:1372–82.

[18] Ejeskär A. Upper limb surgical rehabilitation in high-level tetraplegia. Hand Clin 1988;4:585–99.

[19] Freehafer AA. Gaining independence in tetraplegia. Cleveland technique. Clin Orthop 1998;355:282–9.

[20] Paul SD, Gellman H, Waters R, et al. Single-stage reconstruction of key pinch and extension of the elbow in tetraplegic patients. J Bone Joint Surg 1994; 76A:1451–6.

[21] House JH, Comadoll J, Dahl AL. One-stage key pinch and release with thumb carpal-metacarpal fusion in tetraplegia. J Hand Surg [Am] 1992;17A:530–8.

[22] Meiners T, Abel R, Lindel K, et al. Improvements in activities of daily living following functional hand surgery for treatment of lesions to the cervical spinal cord: self-assessment by patients. Spinal Cord 2002; 40:574–80.

[23] Kiyono Y, Hashizume C, Matsui N, et al. Car-driving abilities of people with tetraplegia. Arch Phys Med Rehabil 2001;82:1389–92.

[24] Kiyono Y, Hashizume C, Ohtsuka K, et al. Improvement of urological-management abilities in individuals with tetraplegia by reconstructive hand surgery. Spinal Cord 2000;38:541–5.

[25] Wuolle KS, Bryden AM, Peckham PH, et al. Satisfaction with upper-extremity surgery in individuals with tetraplegia. Arch Phys Med Rehabil 2003;84:1145–9.

[26] Curtin CM, Gater DR, Chung KC. Upper extremity reconstruction in the tetraplegic population, a national epidemiologic study. J Hand Surg [Am] 2005;30A:94–9.

[27] Curtin CM, Hayward RA, Kim HM, et al. Physician perceptions of upper extremity reconstruction for the person with tetraplegia. J Hand Surg [Am] 2005;30A: 87–93.

The Management of the Upper Limb in Incomplete Lesions of the Cervical Spinal Cord

Vincent R. Hentz, MD[a,b,c,*], Caroline Leclercq, MD[d,e]

[a]Stanford University School of Medicine, Suite 400, 770 Welch Road, Palo Alto, California 94306, USA
[b]Spinal Cord Injury Unit, Veteran Affairs Palo Alto Health Care System, 3801 Miranda Avenue,
Palo Alto, CA 94304, USA
[c]Stanford University Medical Center, Suite 400, 770 Welch Road, Palo Alto, CA 94306, USA
[d]Institut de la Main, Clinique Jouvenet, 6 Square Jouvenet, Paris 75016, France
[e]Centre de Rééducation Neurologique et Fonctionelle, Route de Liverdy, Coubert, France

A complete transection of the spinal cord divides all descending motor tracts as well as all ascending sensory tracts. As a result, paralysis is complete below the lesion. Complete transection also produces a complete sensory loss below the lesion. If the damage occurs at the cervical level, the result is a tetraplegia. Those muscles with motor neurons the level of the spinal lesion are only partially affected. Those muscles with motor neurons above the spinal cord lesion may have fewer than normal motor units, as consequence presumably of the spinal shock accompanying the injury, but otherwise are normal. Those muscles with motor neurons below the spinal cord lesion exhibit the properties of an upper motor neuron paralysis, including exaggerated stretch reflexes and involuntary contractions (spasms), but no voluntary contractions.

In spite of anatomic variation among injured patients, there are sufficient similarities in the clinical presentations of complete injuries at the various cervical spinal cord levels to permit the development and now near universal application of systems of injury classifications, particularly the American Spinal Injury Association (ASIA) classification [1]. The ASIA impairment scale is a modification of the older Frankel [2] scale and assigns patients with spinal cord injuries to one of five categories. In this system, complete lesions are termed ASIA A (complete) and the motor level refers to the most caudal segment of the spinal cord with (preserved) useful motor function. A key muscle (on the right and on the left side of the body) is tested in each of the 10 paired myotomes of the upper and lower limbs. For the upper limb, the key muscles are:

- C5: the elbow flexors (biceps and brachioradialis)
- C6: the wrist extensors (extensor carpi radialis longus and brevis)
- C7: the elbow extensors (triceps)
- C8: the finger flexors (flexor digitorum profundus, middle finger)
- T1: the abductor digiti minimi

The strength of the muscle is graded on a scale of 0 to 5, according to Medical Research Council (MRC) recommendations. The motor level is defined by the lowest key muscle that has a MRC grade of at least 3, provided the key muscles above that level are judged to be normal (grade 4 or 5).

Incomplete lesions of the cervical spinal cord

In contrast, incomplete transection of the spinal cord yields a panoply of postinjury presentations. The ASIA classification scheme includes three categories of incomplete lesions as follows:

B (incomplete): Sensory but not motor function is preserved below the neurologic level and extends through the sacral segments S4-S5.

* Corresponding author. 770 Welch Road, Suite 400, Palo Alto, CA 94304.
E-mail address: vrhentz@stanford.edu (V.R. Hentz).

0749-0712/08/$ - see front matter © 2008 Elsevier Inc. All rights reserved.
doi:10.1016/j.hcl.2008.01.003

C (incomplete): Motor function is preserved below the neurologic level and the majority of key muscles below the neurologic level have a muscle grade less than 3.

D (incomplete): Motor function is preserved below the neurologic level and the majority of key muscles below the neurologic level have a muscle grade greater than or equal to 3.

Spinal cord injury clinical syndromes

Incomplete cord transection is most frequent at the cervical level and results in varied syndromes, depending on the exact site and extent of the lesion. These incomplete syndromes are often much more ill-defined than the complete transection syndrome. However three main syndromes have been characterized: the central (cord) syndrome, the Brown-Sequard syndrome, and the anterior (cord) syndrome (Fig. 1).

The central (cord) syndrome, sometimes referred to as "brachial diplegia," is the most frequently occurring syndrome at the cervical level, accounting for more than half of all incomplete syndromes [3]. It usually results from a hyperextension injury occurring in a rigid, often osteoarthritic spine, which makes it frequent among older tetraplegic patients. The common clinical event is a fall in an elderly individual.

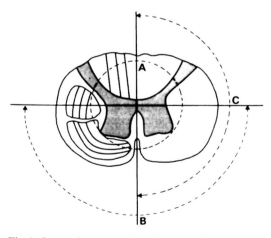

Fig. 1. Incomplete transection of the spinal cord results. (A) Central cord syndrome. (B) Anterior (cord) syndrome. (C) Brown-Sequard syndrome. (*Adapted from* Barat M, Arne I. Les syndromes incompletes [The incomplete syndromes]. In: Maury F, editor. La Paraplegie. Paris: Flammarion; 1981. p. 172–6 [in French]; with permission.)

The cord lesion predominates in the gray matter, extending variably into the white matter [4].

The clinical picture is dominated by a discrepancy between a severe motor loss in the upper limbs and a mild loss in the lower limbs. Lower limbs are almost always involved [5,6]. Clinical findings usually include:

- a flaccid paralysis of the upper limbs, usually including at least two medullary segments
- a spastic and moderate paralysis of the lower limbs
- a dissociated sensory loss, predominating in the thorax and upper limbs, with retained epicritic sensibility and a loss of pain and temperature sensations (analgesia and thermanesthesia).
- retained control of urination and defecation

When the spinal lesion is very limited, the clinical picture may be that of an isolated brachial diplegia. When the lesion is more extensive, the tetraplegia may be subtotal, with only sacral sparing.

Following acute central cord injury, the lower extremities typically recover first, with hand muscle recovering last or not at all. Occasionally, the hands recover but shoulder and elbow muscles do not [7].

The Brown-Sequard syndrome follows a hemisection of the spinal cord. It occurs less than half as often as the central cord syndrome [3]. Very rarely pure, it is often either incomplete or mixed with other neurologic symptoms. It is reported to account for 15% to 20% of incomplete tetraplegia. The causative event is usually a fracture or dislocation in hyperflexion. When pure, it includes:

- a unilateral paralysis of the central type
- an ipsilateral loss of epicritic and deep sensibilities. (The retention of protopathic sensibility produces severe hyperesthesia.)
- an ipsilateral anesthetic zone above the lesion, due to the destruction of the posterior root zone of entry at the level of the damage
- a contralateral dissociated sensory loss, with analgesia and thermanesthesia, but almost normal touch perception

Most of the time, the Brown-Sequard syndrome is partial and mixed, limited to a more severe picture on one side, with a rapid unilateral recovery, and sensory disturbances remaining more important on the side that is recovering.

Brown-Sequard syndromes have the most favorable prognosis of all incomplete lesions because in most cases patients recover the ability to walk and satisfactory bowel and bladder control.

The anterior (cord) syndrome accounts for 25% of incomplete tetraplegias. It can occur as a result of many types of injuries, with a slight predominance of flexion-induced fracture-dislocations of the spine, and of those injuries causing protrusion of the intervertebral disk. The trauma leads to a lesion of the anterior horns and the anterolateral tracts, with a possible division of the anterior spinal artery. The clinical picture includes:

- a flaccid paralysis of the upper limbs, covering several segments
- an initially flaccid paralysis of the lower limbs, with a rapid return of motor reflexes
- a dissociated sensory loss, disproportionate to the motor loss, with analgesia and thermanesthesia, but retained epicritic and deep sensibilities, and with frequent infralesional paresthesias. Lesions at the cervical spine level may be associated with breathing disorders [8].

An isolated lesion of the sulcocommissural arteries results in an ischemia of the anterior horns, with an isolated brachial mono- or diplegia. In a study of 175 patients diagnosed with spinal cord injury clinical syndromes, patients with anterior cord syndromes had the longest hospital stays and the poorest recovery, compared with central cord syndrome or Brown-Sequard syndrome patients [3]. Pollard and Apple [9] retrospectively reviewed 412 patients with traumatic, incomplete cervical spinal cord injuries. When an incomplete cervical spinal cord lesion exists, younger patients and those with either a central cord or Brown-Sequard syndrome have a more favorable prognosis for recovery.

Upper limb evaluation of the patient who has incomplete lesions

For the patient with a cervical spinal cord injury lesion, the focus of the hand surgeon's evaluation has been primarily to classify each limb according to the International Classification system [10] by careful manual muscle testing and standard sensory testing, (eg, two-point discrimination). In general, if the patient has strong (MRC grade 4 or 5) wrist extension, he or she typically possesses strong shoulder abductors, external/internal rotators, and elbow flexion. Joint stiffness may complicate the presentation and

affect function but it is typically the consequence of inattention to or lack of postinjury therapy. For most patients with ASIA A (complete) tetraplegia, once the International Classification level is established, the applicable surgical procedures that might potentially enhance upper limb function can be determined readily, the other essentials of surgical decision-making being present (eg, neurologic and psychologic stability). The same is also true for most patients with ASIA B (incomplete) tetraplegia, who, while they may retain sensation below the cord lesion, have absent motor function below the cord lesion, and also for many ASIA C (incomplete) tetraplegics because retained motor function below the cord lesion is only to an MRC grade 1 or 2 level. In contrast, patients with ASIA D (incomplete) tetraplegia retain MRC grade 3 or greater strength in at least a few or even many muscles innervated distal to the cord lesion. It is difficult to assign easily an International Classification to these patients other than International Classification level X (others). This International Classification does not assist the surgeon in surgical planning to the same extent as the other classifications in this system. For example, we have evaluated four patients who were classified as C-7 ASIA D (incomplete) tetraplegia. Our examination would have resulted in them being assigned an International Classification of CuO:5 (+triceps) except for the presence of a MRC Grade 4 adductor pollicis muscle.

The hand surgeon must be aware of both the patient's ASIA classification before commencing the upper limb examination and also the significance to the examination process for the patient who carries one of the cord syndrome states discussed above. It is our experience that patients with incomplete tetraplegia, especially more severely injured patients, exhibit the following pathologic features far more frequently than patients with complete injuries: upper limb hypertonicity/spasticity; persistent and frequently painful contractures of shoulders, elbows, wrists, and digits; painful hyperesthesias; and paralyzed proximal upper extremity muscles with distal muscle sparing.

Upper limb hypertonicity/spasticity

While a patient with complete lesions may exhibit troublesome and potentially disabling lower limb spasticity, disabling upper limb spasticity is unusual. Patients with incomplete lesions frequently exhibit both troublesome and potentially useful upper limb hypertonicity or frank spasticity. These patients require a more careful motor analysis to identify hypertonic or spastic muscles. Some exhibit hypertonicity in elbow flexors or shoulder adductors that prevents them from reaching out into space. Other patients may be able to trigger a spasm of, for example, their spastic flexor pollicis longus, and achieve a functional grip. Others exhibit persistently extended digits, particularly the index finger, and thus cannot take advantage of tenodesis-derived grip functions.

Persistent and frequently painful contractures of shoulders, elbows, wrists, and digits

These contractures frequently resist standard therapeutic interventions, such as passive range-of-motion exercises. Exercise causes pain and triggers additional hypertonicity, resulting in a vicious spiral leading to a frozen shoulder or elbow. These limbs mimic in many ways the limbs of the poststroke patient, except that they are usually the source of significant pain.

Those patients with central cord syndrome commonly have many muscles that have suffered a flaccid paralysis. The term is somewhat of a misnomer because these lower motor neuron paralyzed muscles don't remain soft or loose, but rather frequently undergo fibrosis and shortening. If the finger flexors are involved, the shortening results in fixed flexion deformities of the digits and, in time, flexion contractures first of the proximal interphalangeal (PIP) joints and then, if severe, contractures of the metacarpophalangeal (MP) joints. A key step in the examination of these patients is to determine if the contracted fingers are a consequence of both shortened, fibrotic muscles and secondary periarticular joint fibrosis, or whether, through exercise, the joints have remained supple. This requires flexing the wrist fully to relax the shortened flexor muscles, and then flexing fully the MP joints and then judging whether, with these maneuvers, the PIP joints can be straightened passively. If the PIP joint cannot be straightened passively, in spite of attempts to slacken the muscle-tendon unit, then both the shortened muscle and the contracted joint will require attention before any functional surgery can be considered.

Painful hyperesthesias

When sensory sparing is present, there may be functionally disabling hyperesthesias in key structures, such as the thumb. Even if greater potential function could be achieved by tenodeses or tendon transfers, these patients would still be unable to use their surgically enhanced grip or pinch because the hypersensitivity persists.

The less severely injured patient may present with a monoplegia characterized by severe compromise of one limb and almost normal retained function of the opposite limb. Some of these patients are completely or almost completely ambulatory and are functioning at a very high level.

Paralyzed proximal upper extremity muscles with distal muscle sparing

Some patients may have preserved finger and thumb flexion and extension but have paralyzed or very weak shoulder muscles. They are able to hold objects in their hand but cannot move the limb to acquire objects, or move acquired objects in a useful way.

Surgical rehabilitation in the complete lesion: a well-established philosophy

To date, most published reports dealing with surgical rehabilitation of the upper limb in patients with tetraplegia have focused on patients with complete transection of the cervical spinal cord [11,12]. For example, the commonly used International Classification system [10] is based on observations of many patients with ASIA A (complete) lesions, ones whose still-functioning muscles, though possessing less than full strength, still respond much like normal muscles. That is, they possess appropriate stretch reflexes and more or less normal patterns of excitation and recruitment. Such muscles, if of sufficient strength, can be transferred reliably to perform a more important functional task. For example, to restore finger flexion and thus grasp, the extensor carpi radialis longus can be transferred to activate the flexor digitorum profundus tendons. The same is true for most ASIA B (incomplete) tetraplegic patients.

Surgery for the upper limb in ASIA C and D (incomplete) lesions: why they may not be good surgical candidates

In contrast to the circumstances for the tetraplegic patient with a complete injury, where there are clearly established benchmark procedures for the various International Classification categories, the surgeon cannot employ such a "recipelike" approach to the patient with an incomplete lesion. A far more individualized approach is needed.

Decisions are more difficult to make and, unfortunately, must be based more on experience than on texts or journals. For example, for patients with complete injuries, muscle-tendon transfers have become the mainstay of reconstruction because the results are relatively predictable. In contrast, it has become an important and well-established surgical axiom that muscles lacking normal excitation parameters perform unreliably if surgically transferred. Therefore, those procedures proven reliable and possible for patients with complete lesions, such as muscle-tendon transfers, may not be so readily adapted to the patient with a severe but still incomplete lesion. Far more often than the completely injured patient, the incompletely injured patient may require preliminary (to the procedures to restore function) therapy or surgery to correct, if possible, the consequences of the injury, especially joint contractures. Paradoxically, the complex problems of the hands and arms of these patients, while requiring far more study and analysis, are best managed by the axiom "keep it simple." The more severely injured of these patients may not respond well to complicated multistage reconstructive surgeries. Simple, more predictable procedures, such as arthrodeses and tenodeses, may be best.

There are other features that complicate surgical decision-making. For the completely injured patient, the usual recommendation is to operate on the arm with the greatest functional potential with the goal of making the operated arm the dominant limb. Some incompletely injured syndromic patients have an almost normal upper limb on one side and are already functioning at a high level (eg, completely independent in all of their activities of daily living). The goal for these patients with essentially a monoplegia is to make the lesser arm somewhat more functional. These patients appropriately question the value of surgery for their affected limb. Paradoxically, by virtue of having an essentially normal arm, they are actually far less inconvenienced by the period of postoperative immobilization and rehabilitation than patients with a complete injury. In a similar analogy, because some of these patients are already fully or partly ambulatory, and don't have to push a wheelchair, they are far less bothered by having the operated "bad" hand in a cast than the completely injured tetraplegic patient who typically requires a power chair during the postoperative period and beyond. Finally, there might not be the same level of motivation and dedication following surgery when the goal is only to improve somewhat the lesser limb.

The surgical armamentarium in the patient who has a severe incomplete lesion

Management of spasticity

Spasticity is a frequent consequence of incomplete injuries. As discussed above, spasticity is a complicating factor in developing a rehabilitation plan. Most often it degrades function, but occasionally patients learn how to control their spasticity in a functionally beneficial manner. Careful analysis of the location and effect of spastic muscles usually suggests a plan for management.

The principal treatments for troublesome spasticity include an initial trial of therapy followed by systemic or localized pharmacologic intervention. Initially, nonpharmacologic physical modalities, including heat, cold, massage, manipulation, and electrical stimulation, should be tried. If nonpharmacologic physical modalities are unsuccessful, oral medications may be tried. These include gamma-aminobutyric acid B receptor agonists, such as baclofen or gabapentin; long-acting benzodiazepines, such as clonazepam; and anticonvulsant agents. Systemic medications, such as baclofen, are usually prescribed initially in gradually increasing doses. Spacticity uncontrolled by systemic medication may respond to more targeted therapy because these same agents may be administered intrathecally by injection or by indwelling catheters and drug pumps. If specific spastic or hypertonic muscles are the cause of disabling limb posture, or are restricting the effectiveness of other therapies, such a joint range-of-motion exercises, then even more targeted therapy is warranted. Therapeutic modalities include intramuscular (motor-point) injection of short- or long-acting local anesthetics or peripheral nerve blocks with local anesthetics or with longer-acting neurotoxic agents. Phenol or alcohol have long been used [13,14]. They are not reliably reversible and should be used with great discretion and then only following a therapeutic trial with a long-acting local anesthetic agent, such as bupivacaine. Their use in incomplete spinal cord lesions may lead to impaired recovery and diminished ultimate function. In addition, the long-term response has been suboptimal. Braun [15] reports only 4 of 15 patients had an acceptable long-term response to phenol blockade.

The goal is to weaken or paralyze the overactive muscle or muscles so that weakened antagonist muscles, if under neural control, might be exercised to become more functional. A second, more common goal is to enhance the effectiveness of conventional treatments for shortened muscles or contracted joints, such as serial casting, dynamic splinting, and joint ranging.

The bacterium clostridium botulinum produces a toxin that causes flaccid paralysis of muscles by interfering with acetylcholine release. It has gained wide use as a means of controlling spasticity because its effect is essentially completely reversible within 2 to 3 months following injection. It has been used with success in C5/6 tetraplegia to block spastic forearm muscles [16,17]. Currently, the injection of botulinum toxin (Botox) into hyperactive or spastic muscles has become the preferred treatment. We have had a positive experience with Botox injections into hypertonic shoulder adductors and in particular into spastic elbow flexors, usually guided by electrical stimulation. The treated muscle will regain its innervation but occasionally it is less spastic upon recovery. The most important benefit from such procedures is that the immediate reduction in flexor spasticity allows the therapist to be more effective in overcoming muscle shortening and early contractures. We have on occasion, by preliminary electromyographic analysis, identified the biceps as spastic while the brachialis muscle was much less so. In this case, Botox injection into the biceps muscle eliminated functionally troublesome elbow flexor spasticity, yet did not significantly weaken elbow flexion. This allowed the patient some useful elbow flexor strength. Fig. 2 illustrates the benefit of Botox in relieving troublesome spasticity and enhancing function. The patient is a 36-year-old man with C6 ASIA C (incomplete) tetraplegia whose spasticity restricted his ability to reach out into space and acquire objects. Dynamic electromyographic analysis (A–C) demonstrated cocontracture of biceps and triceps muscles as he attempted to extend his elbow and reach for an object. He had injections of Botox into hypertonic biceps and finger flexors. His pre-Botox (D and F) and post-Botox (E and G) posture is illustrated. Injections frequently need to be repeated, but we have noted in a few cases a reduction in muscle hypertonicity that persists long after the expected pharmacologic activity of the Botox has ceased.

Other surgical procedures to control spasticity or hyperactive muscles include total or partial neurectomy. We have had some experience in patients with incomplete lesions who present with troublesome intrinsic muscle hypertonicity or spasticity and who have developed a flexion contracture of the MP joints and an adducted thumb not amenable to therapy. Botox injections may produce some level of temporary improvement but it's difficult to inject accurately into the many interosseous muscles. In such cases, we have performed a selective neurectomy of the motor branch of the ulnar nerve. This has allowed the therapist to be more successful in restoring some MP joint flexibility. Selective partial neurectomy at the level of the motor plate (terminal ending of the nerve into the muscle fibers), termed hyponeurotization, is usually preceded by Botox injections to assess the potential effectiveness of a permanent decrease of spasticity. It is usually quite effective in large single-body muscles. It may, however, require an extensive surgical exposure, as is the case, for example, with hyperactive finger flexor muscles.

Tendon transfers

Even though the outcome of tendon transfers may be less predictable in this population, tendon transfers may be useful. The surgeon should be confident that the muscle to be transferred is of sufficient power and under good voluntary control. It is important to review the history of recovery of muscles in these patients. For example, a muscle that had no movement for months following injury but has instead very slowly, perhaps over years, recovered strength to an MRC grade 4 level is, in our opinion, an unreliable muscle for tendon transfer. We have seen such muscles lose essentially all their preoperative power following transfer. For such patients, there may be a role for a detailed electrophysiological evaluation of the proposed muscle. If the muscle shows evidence of abnormal regeneration (eg, persistently huge motor units on electromyographic testing), it will probably perform poorly if transferred. We hypothesize that some of these muscles experienced a concomitant major lower motor palsy, are at best regenerated muscles, and, as such, are notably poor performers following tendon transfer.

Because many of these patients may exhibit a flaccid (lower motor neuron) paralysis over several medullary segments, some muscles become fibrotic and frequently foreshortened, even if they are not causing a joint contracture. At the time of

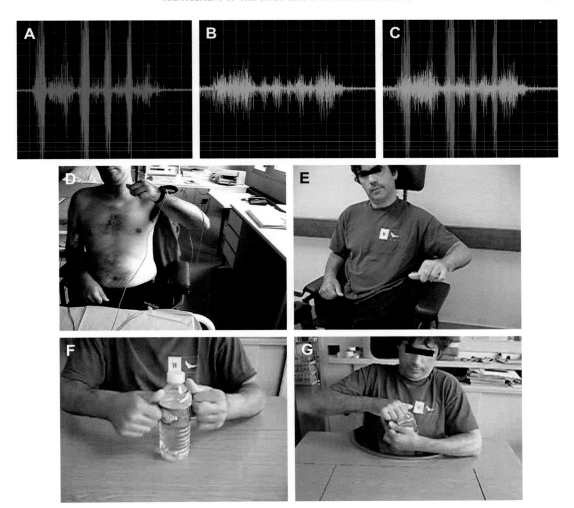

Fig. 2. Preinjection dynamic electromyogram performed while patient was trying to extend the elbow. Electromyogram recorded from biceps (*A*) and triceps (*B*) and superimposed (*C*). Pre-Botox injection shoulder and elbow posture (*D*) and postinjection posture (*E*). Pre-Botox injection hand posture (*F*) and postinjection posture (*G*).

tendon transfer, it is wise to excise a segment of the paralyzed muscle just proximal to the point where its tendon becomes the recipient for the tendon transfer. This step decreases the possibility of the fibrotic muscle interfering with excursion of the recipient tendon following transfer. The same applies when transferring a muscle to another spastic one: Sectioning the recipient muscle proximal to the suture site alleviates the spastic component.

We have performed surgery for the poor arm in four ambulatory patients with probable Brown-Sequard syndrome and monoplegia, although two patients may have had some element of a brachial plexus injury as well as a spinal cord injury. Two

patients had their involved limb classified as CuO:5 but with 3+ digital extensor strength and some preservation of function of the abductor pollicis brevis. Both had two-stage grasp release procedures. In the first stage, an MRC grade 3+ or 4− flexor carpi ulnaris was transferred into the extensor digitorum communis and to rerouted extensor pollicis longus tendons to augment digital extension, and the split flexor pollicis longus (FPL) was transferred to the extensor pollicis longus to stabilize the thumb interphalangeal joint. This was followed some weeks later by transfer of the extensor carpi radialis longus to the flexor digitorum profundus (FDP) tendons and the transfer of brachioradialis to the FPL. Both patients recovered useful helping hand function in the operated limb (Fig. 3). We transferred the extensor carpi radialis longus to the FDP and the brachioradialis to the FPL in a third ambulatory patient who requested surgery to improve a weak grip and pinch for his poor arm. His grip strength of 30 N before surgery increased to 60 N following surgery.

Tenotomies/muscle-tendon lengthening and capsulotomies

Patients with a complete injury may experience tightness in hypertonic or spastic muscle groups. The muscle shortened because of increased tone responds to nerve blocks or injections of botulinum toxin to diminish tone. Once tone is

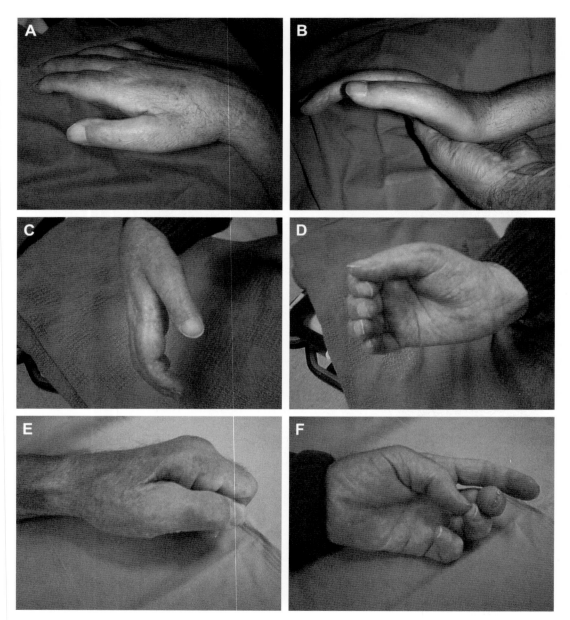

Fig. 3. Preoperative aspect of the "poor" hand with wrist flexion (*A*) and wrist extension (*B*). Postoperative appearance following multiple tendon transfers for pinch and grip (*C–F*). See text for operative details.

diminished, passive stretching may relieve the contracture. In contrast, in many incomplete lesions, flaccid paralyses frequently predominate. Therapy rarely overcomes the contracture if these muscles become fibrotic and contracted. Tenotomy or tendon lengthening procedures are generally needed to overcome contractures.

We have treated several patients with central cord syndrome who have developed severe claw deformities with fixed extension contractures of the MP joints. Fig. 4 shows the hand of such a patient. He was classified according to the International Classification system as CuO:X because of the unusual pattern of muscles still under some voluntary control. For example, he had MRC grade 4 radial wrist extension and MRC grade 4 finger flexors but no active digital extension or wrist flexion. We felt that he was a candidate for creation of a key pinch procedure as described by Moberg [12]. However, his MP hyperextension

contracture would have made it impossible for him to have a stable platform for pinching. In addition, he had relatively limited shoulder and elbow range and would have found it nearly impossible to roll his fingers into flexion in preparation for key pinch with the thumb, even in the absence of contracted MP joints. We chose to perform a preliminary MP joint dorsal capsulotomy with judicious and minimal division of collateral ligaments. This allowed us to manipulate his MP joints into flexion. Each MP joint was pinned in flexion with a Kirschner wire that was removed after 4 weeks. We chose to allow these joints to stiffen somewhat in a flexed posture and in a position that would permit a stable key pinch. Several months later, we performed a key pinch procedure. Following surgery, he achieved a weak but still functionally useful key grip that allowed him to eat with minimal set-up assistance (Fig. 4B–D).

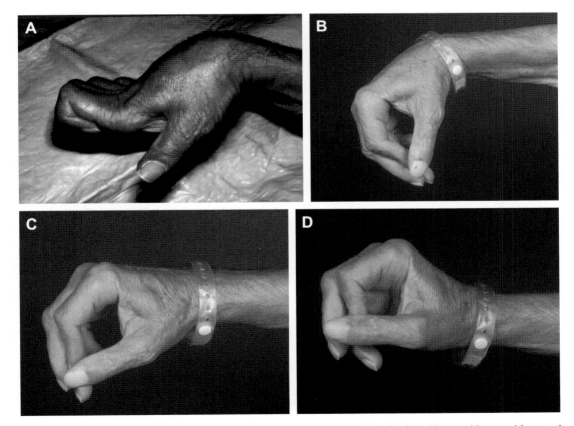

Fig. 4. Preoperative appearance (*A*) demonstrating fixed hyperextension deformity in a 65-year-old man with central cord syndrome. Postoperative appearance (*B–D*) following initial MP joint capsulotomy, tendon lengthening, and subsequent key pinch procedure.

Tenodeses

Many patients with incomplete cervical spinal cord lesions are able to ambulate, either with assistance or unassisted. They do not need to "walk" on their hands and, therefore, they do not have the constant stresses of weight-bearing on their hands as do patients with complete lesions. In these patients, a tenodesis, when appropriate, will not be at the same risk of stretching over time.

Arthrodeses

Because fused joints are not expected to be subject to the same level of stress in the ambulatory patient, joints in ambulating patients with incomplete injuries may, when appropriate, be arthrodesed safely in positions that would not be appropriate for the patient who must "walk" on his or her hands. For example, the thumb's carpometacarpal (CMC) joint can be arthrodesed in a somewhat more palmarly abducted position to achieve a more precise termino-terminal or three-point tip-to-tip pinch. The authors typically avoid this widely abducted position when arthrodesing the CMC joint of a tetraplegic patient, because the widely abducted thumb interferes with transfers and with motions required for propelling the wheelchair. Experience has taught the authors that, if this joint is arthrodesed in too much palmar abduction, the fusion may over time break down.

Summary

Patients who have incomplete cervical spinal cord injuries present unique challenges for the reconstructive surgeon. For example:

- Their patterns of injury don't easily fit into the International Classification system familiar to surgeons.
- They don't lend themselves to a "recipe" approach to surgical decision-making.
- They frequently have developed upper limb deformities that must be addressed before any consideration is made for functional surgery.
- Little regarding surgery for these patients has been published.

While challenging, many patients who have incomplete cervical spine injuries benefit by comprehensive evaluation and carefully planned surgical procedures.

References

[1] American Spinal Injury Association. Standards for neurological and functional classification of spinal cord injury. Atlanta (GA): American Spinal Injury Association; 1992.

[2] Frankel HL, Hancock DO, Hyslop G, et al. The value of postural reduction in the initial management of closed injuries of the spine with paraplegia and tetraplegia. Paraplegia 1969;7:179–92.

[3] McKinley W, Santos K, Meade M, et al. Incidence and outcomes of spinal cord injury clinical syndromes. J Spinal Cord Med 2007;30(3):215–24.

[4] Fuentes JM, Vlahovitch B, Nègre C. Central Cord Syndrome [Brachial diplegia of traumatic origin as a result of injuries of the cervical cord]. Neurochirurgie 1984;30(3):165–70 [in French].

[5] Rajabally YA, Hbahbih M, Messios N, et al. Brachial diplegia as a result of cervical cord injury. Spinal Cord 2005;43(6):389–91.

[6] Dai L, Jia L. Acute central cervical cord injury presenting with only upper extremity involvement. Int Orthop 1997;21(6):380–2.

[7] Borovich B, Peyser E, Gruskiewicz J. Acute central and intermediate cervical cord injury. Neurochirurgia (Stuttg) 1978;21(3):77–84.

[8] Manconi M, Mondini S, Fabiani A, et al. Anterior spinal artery syndrome complicated by the ondine curse. Arch Neurol 2003;60(12):1787–90.

[9] Pollard ME, Apple DF. Factors associated with improved neurologic outcomes in patients with incomplete tetraplegia. Spine 2003;28(1):33–9.

[10] McDowell CL, Moberg EA, Graham Smith A. International conference on surgical rehabilitation of the upper limb in tetraplegia. J Hand Surg [Am] 1979;4:387–90.

[11] Hentz V, Leclercq C. Surgical rehabilitation of the upper limb in tetraplegia. London: W.B. Saunders; 2002.

[12] Moberg E. Surgical treatment for absent single-hand grip and elbow extension in quadriplegia: principles and preliminary treatment. J Bone Joint Surg Am 1975;57(2):196–206.

[13] Khalili AA, Harmel MH, Forster S, et al. Management of spasticity by selective periphereal nerve block with dilute phenol solutions in clinical rehabilitation. Arch Phys Med Rehabil 1964;45:513–9.

[14] Wainapel SF, Haigney D, Labib K. Spastic hemiplegia in a quadriplegic patient: treatment with phenol nerve block. Arch Phys Med Rehabil 1984;65:786–7.

[15] Braun RM, Hoffer MM, Mooney V, et al. Phenol nerve block in treatment of acquired spastic hemiplegia in upper limb. J Bone Joint Surg 1973;55:580–5.

[16] Cromwell SJ, Paquette V. The effect of botulinum toxin A on the function of a person with poststroke quadriplegia. Phys Ther 1996;76:395–402.

[17] Richardson D, Sheean G, Greenwood R, et al. The effect of botulinum toxin on hand function after complete spinal cord injury at the level of C5/6. Clin Rehabil 1997;11(4):288–92.

Reconstruction of Elbow Extension

Caroline Leclercq, MD[a,b,*], Vincent R. Hentz, MD[c,d,e],
Scott H. Kozin, MD[f,g], Mary Jane Mulcahey, PhD, OTR/L[h]

[a]Institut de la Main, Clinique Jouvenet, 6 Square Jouvenet, Paris 75016, France
[b]Centre de Rééducation Neurologique et Fonctionnelle, Route de Liverdy, Coubert, France
[c]Stanford University School of Medicine, Suite 400, 770 Welch Road, Palo Alto, California 94306, USA
[d]Spinal Cord Injury Unit, Veterans Affairs Palo Alto Health Care System, 3801 Miranda Avenue,
Palo Alto, CA 94304, USA
[e]Stanford University Medical Center, Suite 400, 770 Welch Road, Palo Alto, CA 94306, USA
[f]Department of Orthopaedic Surgery, Temple University, 3401 North Broad Street, Philadelphia, PA 19140, USA
[g]Pediatric Hand and Upper Extremity Center of Excellence, Shriners Hospitals for Children,
3551 North Broad Street, Philadelphia, PA 19140, USA
[h]Shriners Hospital for Children, 3551 North Broad Street, Philadelphia, PA 19140, USA

Patients in a wheelchair use their upper limbs to propel the chair. Without triceps function, they cannot "push through" with a full motion. This deficit makes pushing a wheelchair less efficient and more energy consuming, restricting the wheelchair "environment" to level ground. Most tetraplegic patients who lack triceps function ultimately turn to a powered chair despite the disadvantages of such chairs, that is, their cost, increased size, and weight.

When seated in a wheelchair, the reach of the tetraplegic patient is determined by the range of motion of his or her upper extremities. The world that lies beyond the patient's immediate reach can be acquired only be moving the wheelchair to position the object to be acquired closer to the individual. Without the ability to extend the elbow, the patient's functional environment is much reduced. The ability to extend the hand away from the body by an additional 12 in results in an additional 800% of space that the hand can reach. Because of the patient's sitting and lower position, many of the objects that he or she needs to reach, such as door knobs, light switches, and elevator buttons, are located above the level of the shoulders. Without active elbow extension, these objects are beyond reach.

Tetraplegic patients spend many hours in bed. When the patient is lying supine, his or her hands frequently fall into the face without active elbow extension when trying to reach overhead. In spinal cord injury at the C5-C6 level, C5 innervated muscles such as the deltoid and biceps-brachialis may function sufficiently for the patient to have good shoulder control and strong elbow flexion; however, elbow flexion may be unopposed because the triceps muscle is paralyzed. This situation may lead to the development of a dysfunctional flexion contracture of the elbow.

There are other reasons why reconstruction of active elbow extension is tremendously useful. Without active elbow extension, the tetraplegic patient must learn various adaptive maneuvers to lift their thighs and buttocks to relieve the effects of pressure caused by sitting on these tissues. If the elbows retain full passive extension, the patient may be able to lock the elbows in full or slight hyperextension and, by leaning forward, perform effective pressure relief; however, if the trunk is unstable, the patient may pitch forward. With active elbow extension, the tetraplegic patient can more easily perform pressure relief maneuvers and reduce the risk of developing ischial or sacral pressure sores. This same ability allows the tetraplegic patient to assist his or her caregiver in safely performing transfers from

---

* Corresponding author. Institut de la Main, 6 Square Jouvenet, Paris 75016, France.
  E-mail address: caroline.leclercq@free.fr
(C. Leclercq).

0749-0712/08/$ - see front matter © 2008 Elsevier Inc. All rights reserved.
doi:10.1016/j.hcl.2008.02.003

a bed to chair or from a chair to a toilet. Even a relatively small elbow extension torque, much less than that required to reach high over head or to propel a manual chair up a gradient and far below that needed to self-transfer, will be of major functional significance if controllable. This small extension torque may allow the patient to control the arm as he or she reaches out into space or to accurately direct the arm to the target in a controlled and coordinated manner versus having to launch the arm in the general direction of the target. With a small amount of elbow extensor power, patients do not need to depend solely on the braking function of their elbow flexors in controlling the trajectory and velocity of their arms in space. Restoring this critical element of control may be the most beneficial aspect of reconstruction of elbow extension.

Surgical techniques for restoring active elbow extension

Two surgical procedures are advocated for restoring active elbow extension— transfer of a strong portion of the deltoid muscle into the triceps and transfer of the biceps muscle into the triceps. Each of these techniques has strong advocates and opponents.

Instead of championing either one of these techniques, the intent of this article is to describe each procedure fully by a regular user (deltoid to triceps [CL and VRH]; biceps to triceps [SK and MJM]), along with providing detailed indications, contraindications, and reasons for preference.

Part one: deltoid to triceps transfer

The synergism between the posterior part of the deltoid and the triceps muscle was recognized by Merle d'Aubigne and colleagues [1] who suggested that the posterior half of the deltoid might substitute for the paralyzed triceps. Moberg [2] was the first to establish that this transfer could provide predictable elbow extension power in the tetraplegic patient.

Indication and contraindications

Absolute contraindications include fixed elbow flexion contracture and inadequate strength of the posterior half of the deltoid muscle. If the elbow is contracted in a flexed posture, the flexion contracture should be treated by progressive splinting or dynamic stretching. If these conservative measures fail and elbow flexion contracture remains greater than 45 degrees, surgical release before

deltoid to triceps transfer should be performed, or a biceps to triceps transfer should be advocated.

A careful determination of the strength of the posterior part of the deltoid must be performed before deciding on the choice of technique. This determination can be performed in two manners as follows:

> With the patient sitting in their wheelchair, the observer stands behind the arm to be tested. The patient is then advised to loop the elbow of the opposite arm around the handle of the wheelchair to stabilize the trunk. The patient is asked first to horizontally abduct the arm to 90 degrees of abduction (which automatically flexes the elbow nearly completely) and then to push as hard as possible against the observer's palm placed against the posterior surface of the patient's humerus. The tension and mass of the posterior half of the deltoid is assessed by the observer's opposite hand grasping the muscle as the patient makes a maximal effort. If the patient's arm can be easily pushed out of the extended position, the strength of the posterior part of the deltoid is probably insufficient to permit a predictable outcome after surgery.
>
> The same maneuver is effected with the patient lying prone, the shoulder resting on the edge of the examination table, and the arm abducted to 90 degrees (Fig. 1).

If the posterior part of the deltoid measured in either of these two manners is rated less than 4 in the Medical Research Council (MRC) classification, it should not be used as a transfer to restore elbow extension.

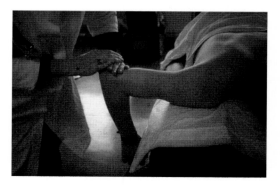

Fig. 1. Testing the strength of the deltoid muscle. The patient pushes his elbow as hard as possible on the hand of the observer.

Relative contraindications are associated with the particular rehabilitative regimen following this surgery. The 4-week postsurgery period of immobilization in a long-arm cast is followed by an even longer interval of directed exercise and the continuous wearing of an orthotic device. This rigorous rehabilitation schedule is a significant challenge for the tetraplegic patient. Deltoid to triceps transfer surgery should be approached with caution if there are questions about the patient's ability to participate fully in this vigorous and relatively complex rehabilitation process.

Surgical technique

The procedure is usually performed under general anesthesia or a supraclavicular brachial plexus block. Allieu and colleagues [3] has pioneered performing this procedure under cervical epidural anesthesia in the tetraplegic patient. The patient may be positioned laterally or in a prone position. The anterior and lateral shoulder and the entire arm are draped free for exposure.

Surgical landmarks at the level of the shoulder include the tip of the acromion superiorly, the interval between the posterior margin of the deltoid and the triceps muscle posteriorly, and the estimated point of insertion of the deltoid on the humerus distally. Landmarks at the level of the elbow include the tip of the olecranon and the insertion of the triceps tendon (Fig. 2). The surgeon should keep in mind the neurovascular anatomy of the region, including the course of the axillary nerve and the circumflex humeral artery and the radial nerve and its relationship to the insertion of the deltoid.

The upper incision is centered halfway between the midaxial line of the humerus and the posterior margin of the deltoid. The skin incision is carried to the level of the muscle fascia, and the skin and subcutaneous tissue are elevated anteriorly as far as the anterior margin of the deltoid muscle. Posteriorly, the skin flap is elevated to the margin of deltoid and the long head of the triceps (Fig. 3). The plane between these two muscles is developed by sharp or finger dissection. The interval is relatively bloodless and easily dissected. A finger will slip under the deltoid muscle at about the midportion of this muscle. It is insinuated through the fibers of the muscle, separating off the posterior half. The fibers of the deltoid are split in the direction of the muscle fascicles by blunt dissection.

The posterior half of the muscle is then detached from its point of insertion into the humerus by sharply incising a rectangle of the periosteum at the point of attachment and elevating the periosteum in continuity with the fibers of attachment off the humerus. Care is taken to include as much fascia and fibrous insertion as possible, including some of the fascial origin of the brachioradialis muscle. The radial nerve will emerge from behind the humerus several centimeters distal to this point. Injury to this nerve has been reported as a complication of this procedure; therefore, care should be exercised regarding the anatomic landmarks.

A suture is placed in the detached fibrous origin, and dissection of the muscle is carried superiorly (Fig. 4) until the branches of the axillary nerve are visualized. These branches must not be injured, and the superior dissection should stop at this point.

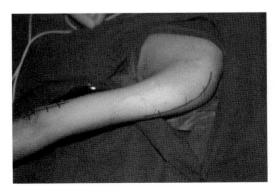

Fig. 2. Skin incisions proximal over the deltoid muscle and distal over the insertion of the triceps tendon (patient lying prone).

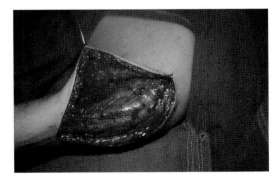

Fig. 3. Elevation of the posterior skin flap to the margin of the deltoid and the long head of the triceps (same patient in Fig. 2).

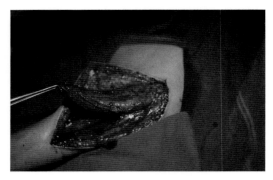

Fig. 4. Elevation of the posterior deltoid from distal to proximal until the branches of the axillary nerve (same patient in Fig. 2).

Several methods have been proposed to attach the posterior deltoid to the triceps or olecranon employing different tissues or materials. Various pieces of the patient's tendons have been used, including toe extensors (Fig. 5A) [2], tibialis anterior tendon [4], or extensor carpi ulnaris [5]. In another method, a strip of a fascia lata (Fig. 5B) [6] is harvested through several transverse incisions placed over the iliotibial band with a fascial stripper. It is tubed about the fibrous insertion of the deltoid and tunneled subcutaneously to the olecranon. The fascia lata is then separated into two tails which are inserted into each end of an oblique tunnel created through the olecranon. The two fascia lata tails are pulled to tense the transfer and anchored to the fascia lata tube with nonabsorbable sutures.

A turned up strip of the central part of the triceps tendon [7] including synthetic reinforcement [8] and measuring 1.5 cm can be harvested in continuity with a periosteal flap from the ulna and then turned superiorly. The deltoid is detached from the humerus along with a periosteal flap. The two fresh periosteal flaps are sutured to each other. The surgeon then buries the tendon reflected and all reinforcing material within the substance of the muscle itself. A modification of this technique (Fig. 5C) [9] uses a bone-to-bone juncture between a segment of the humerus with deltoid attachment and a segment of olecranon harvested in continuity with a central strip of triceps tendon.

Various synthetic materials have also been used [3]. The first author (CL) currently uses a synthetic funnel-shaped Dacron graft designed by Jacques Tessier from France (Fig. 6A). The proximal funnel is sutured around the distal origin of the muscle with nonabsorbable braided sutures anchored to the strong fibrous fibers of the muscle, which are located posteriorly. The graft is then passed subcutaneously to the dorsum of the elbow and its two tails woven into the terminal tendon of the triceps (Fig. 6B).

Postoperative regimen

The elbow is immobilized in full extension using a light fiberglass cylinder cast. The shoulder is kept somewhat abducted, and the patient and other caregivers are cautioned to not allow the shoulder to accidentally flop across the chest. The patient is encouraged to begin getting into his or her wheelchair on the second postoperative day. A sling is fitted to the wheelchair, holding the arm somewhat abducted from the body in a position that relaxes the deltoid.

The cast is removed about 4 weeks after surgery. Other authorities recommend longer periods of casting [10]. The patient begins active exercises in a protective polyaxial brace that limits the amount of flexion but permits full extension (Fig. 7). This active brace is worn essentially full time during the day and blocked in full extension at night.

Exercises are initiated about the fifth postoperative week. Typically, the patient begins attempts to trigger the transfer while the arm is supported in a horizontal, gravity eliminate position. As time passes, the patient tries to trigger the transfer against gravity but without any additional resistance. Resistance exercises are avoided for 8 weeks. The degree of flexion allowed is gradually increased by increments of 10 to 15 degrees per week until the elbow reaches 90 degrees of flexion. The dynamic brace can be abandoned at this time. The patient avoids resistance activities such as transferring on the extended elbow for at least 10 weeks. He or she is encouraged to start leisure activities that require active elbow extension, such as swimming (back stroke), table tennis, and weaving (Fig. 8).

Some months of cautious use are necessary to prevent overstretching of the transfer, and many months pass before maximal strength is obtained.

Outcome of deltoid to triceps transfers
Authors' series. The authors have experience with 83 deltoid to triceps transfers in 56 patients. The results have been fairly consistent, with the great majority of patients achieving full or near full extension against gravity. A few patients are able to fully extend the elbow in the completely overhead posture (Fig. 9). Almost all have gained the ability to better control the elbow, allowing them

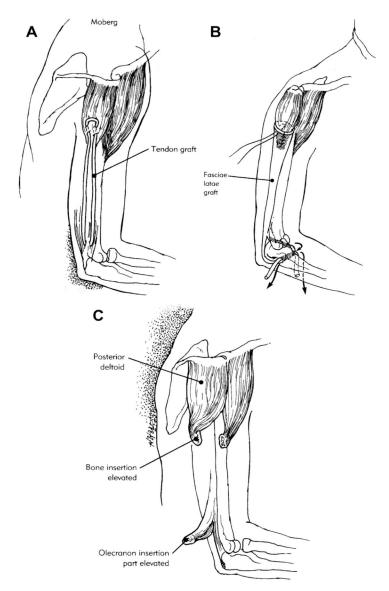

Fig. 5. Various methods of attaching the posterior deltoid to the elbow. (*A*) Toe extensor grafts (Moberg). (*B*) A strip of fascia lata (Hentz). (*C*) A strip of triceps tendon with a segment of olecranon and a bone-to-bone juncture (Castro-Serra and Lopez-Pita). (*From* Hentz VR, Leclercq C. Surgical rehabilitation of the upper limb in tetraplegia. London: Saunders; 2002. p. 105; with permission.)

to more accurately position their arm in space and control its movements.

Functionally, the majority find that they achieve more efficient transfers, pressure releases, and wheelchair mobility. Other functional gains include the ability to reach distant objects, including overhead, ease of turning in bed, improved writing ability, and an improved ability to groom, feed, and drive an automobile (Fig. 10). One patient achieved little useful function following his initial procedure. The transfer was tightened at a second procedure without much improvement.

The authors have not been able to correlate preoperative deltoid strength with the level of final elbow extension torque. Other groups have reported similar inconstant results, although

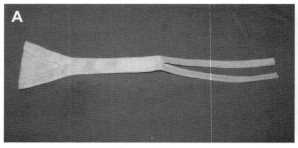
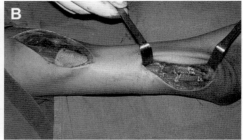

Fig. 6. (*A*) Funnel-shaped Dacron graft. (*B*) The graft is sutured to the deltoid proximally and woven into the triceps distally.

failure of the procedure to provide useful function is rare. Complications are rare provided that the patient follows the exercise protocol and does not overstretch the transfer by performing full elbow flexion too rapidly.

Other series. Moberg [2] reported on his initial 16 patients undergoing deltoid to triceps transfer. Fifteen of the 16 patients experienced significant functional improvement. Two patients experienced overstretching of the transfer. Reoperation with tightening of the transfer in one resulted in satisfactory function. The other patient represents the only failure.

Bryan [11] reported on seven patients who had bilateral transfers, several simultaneously. The results were inconsistent, with some patients demonstrating great postoperative strength and others little strength.

DeBenedetti [12] reported on the outcome of 20 transfers in 17 patients. The average elbow extension strength improved from MRC grade 0.5 (0–2) to grade 3.6 (2.5–4.5) following surgery.

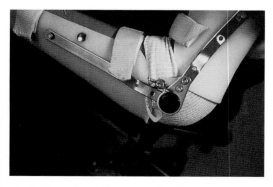

Fig. 7. The polyaxial brace allowing full active extension but limiting flexion.

Using a weight and pulley system, the weight that could be lifted by patients averaged 4.6 lb (range, 1–9 lb). All 13 patients were satisfied with their results, and 11 stated that they would have the procedure again.

Castro-Serra and Lopez-Pita [7] reported the outcomes of 10 elbows in seven patients using their method of tendon attachment. All patients had a satisfactory outcome.

Raczka and colleagues [13] reported the outcomes in a series of 23 transfers in 22 patients. On objective testing, nine patients had gained MRC grade 4 to 4+, four patients MRC grade 3+, and three MRC grade 2+ (but with good functional improvement). Fifteen patients said they had gained functional improvement, including stability of the arm (15), the ability to reach overhead objects (15), turning in bed (10), pressure relief (12), writing (12), driving ability (11), and hygiene skills. Six patients who were not able to drive before surgery were now able to drive. One patient went to a manual chair exclusively. One patient said he was worse because of decreased supination, perhaps secondary to prolonged casting. Initial failures occurred in three patients. There were two failures. In one patient, the original graft failed in its mid substance; in the second patient, the anterior deltoid was secondarily transferred with a gain to MRC grade 2+.

Allieu and colleagues [3] reported the results of their initial 21 cases. They used fascia lata reinforced with Dacron sutures. Although the excursion and power of the transfer was less than expected, subjectively, the results were considered by the patients to be satisfactory despite the inability to actively fully extend the elbow.

Lacey [4] reported the first biomechanical analysis of this transfer. A 5-kg pull was used to stretch the muscle into its full passive length. Then using intraoperative electrical stimulation,

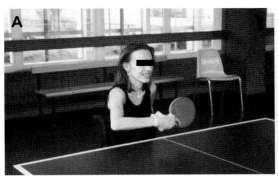
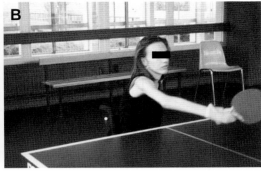

Fig. 8. (*A,B*) Patient exercising her transfer with table tennis. Restoration of hand function will be performed at a later stage.

they determined the excursion of the posterior deltoid to be 7.31 cm. A surprisingly flat and active length-tension curve was measured. Postoperatively, elbow extension torque averaged 36.4 kg-cm (range, 58 to 21 kg-cm). Maximum strength was noted when the elbow was between 30 and 90 degrees of elbow flexion. They noted a large effective range for the deltoid. Clinical results were judged to be excellent in 16 transfers. The average MRC grade was 3 (range, 2–4). They measured 3 cm of excursion in tendon graft to achieve full motion of the elbow, substantially less than that measured for the posterior deltoid. They recommended that tension be adjusted by putting in the distal site first, followed by flexing the elbow to 90 degrees and abducting the shoulder to 30 degrees, and putting the proximal end in while the deltoid is pulled to its normal insertion length.

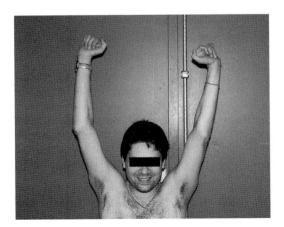

Fig. 9. Satisfactory outcome after bilateral deltoid to triceps transfer at 2 years on the left arm and 5 months on the right arm.

They believe that this positioning maximizes force production in the most useful elbow range.

A later biomechanical study [14] looked at the length-tension relationship of the posterior deltoid to triceps transfer and compared it with the normal triceps. The investigators found that maximum torque was in 130 degrees of elbow flexion, and that normal triceps produced an average of 27 Nm while deltoid to triceps transfer, measured in eight tetraplegic patients, produced 7.8 Nm. They concluded that the initial tension set by the surgeon was the most significant variable and was difficult to control without some type of device dedicated to attaining nominal length-tension relationships.

In 1988, Ejeskar and Dahllof [15] updated the results of reconstruction of elbow extension from Goteborg, Sweden, including Moberg's original operated patients. Between 1970 and 1983, 40 elbows in 32 patients had surgery, 30 by Moberg's method and 10 by the method of Castro-Serra and Lopez-Pita. Eight of the 30 patients undergoing the Moberg method had full extension against gravity, whereas only one of the ten patients undergoing the Castro-Serra method achieved this. Thirteen of the 30 patients undergoing the Moberg method and seven of the ten undergoing the Castro-Serra method had greater than a 60-degree extension lag with the arm overhead but could still control the elbow. Ejeskar advocated placing steel sutures on either side of the tendon junctures to allow an estimation of tendon elongation in the postoperative period.

Mennen and Boonzaier [9] described a modification of the Castro-Serra technique and reported the results in 35 procedures performed since 1983. His patients achieved on average the strongest level of elbow extension torque thus reported.

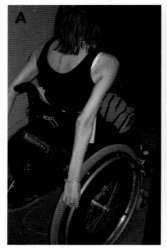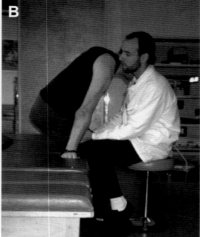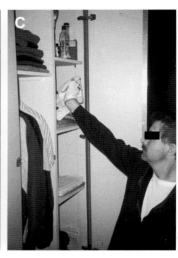

Fig. 10. Functional gains after restoration of active elbow extension by deltoid to triceps transfer. (*A*) More efficient wheelchair mobility, including the ability to reach the wheel posteriorly. (*B*) Pressure release. (*C*) Reaching overhead.

Manual muscle testing (MMT) was performed. Seven patients achieved MRC grade 5 strength, 25 patients achieved grade 4, and three patients achieved grade 3. Three patients were able to perform self-transfers. One patient required re-exploration and was found to have developed a boutonnière deformity of the remaining triceps insertion. This defect was repaired with a good result. One patient suffered a fractured humerus.

Lieber and colleagues [16] measured the extent and timing of elbow extension torque recovery after posterior deltoid to triceps tendon transfer in 40 limbs in 23 patients and performed a comparison with healthy controls and persons with C7 spinal cord injuries. Based on the shape of the moment-joint angle curve and using a biomechanical model, it was predicted that the posterior deltoid was inserted at a relatively short muscle length of 123.1 mm and thus operated exclusively on the ascending limb of the length-tension relationship. These observations suggest that connective tissue septa restrict muscle fiber elongation during surgical tensioning of the tendon transfer, and that this relatively short length would result in a significant force loss should any of the repair sites slip or stretch during rehabilitation.

Hentz and Leclercq [17] has reported the long-term assessment of 45 patients operated on at least 10 years earlier. Of the 21 patients who underwent elbow extensor reconstruction, 15 had posterior deltoid to triceps transfer. All 15 patients had required a motorized wheelchair as their primary means of movement before surgery. Ten years after surgery, nine patients used a manual chair as their standard chair, and four others used a manual chair at least some of the time. Three patients who underwent bilateral posterior deltoid to triceps transfer were able to self-transfer in the early postoperative period. All three continue to be able to perform this task, which is monumental for a tetraplegic patient. Of the six patients having biceps to triceps transfer (all needing contracture release), two can use a manual chair, but not exclusively so.

Discussion

There was initial concern that transferring part of the tetraplegic patient's deltoid muscle might result in functional loss at the shoulder. Such loss has not been found, although few studies have addressed this question by truly quantitative measurements. Simply moving the insertion of the deltoid more distal on the humerus should not change its biomechanical properties relative to its function at the shoulder, except for potentially weakening this part of the muscle by surgical manipulation.

In his 1978 monograph, Moberg [18] reported adding the anterior half of the deltoid to the transfer as a secondary procedure in an attempt to improve elbow extension power or salvage an initial suboptimal outcome. Hentz [17] has reported a similar experience and has not seen changes in postoperative shoulder function following transfer of the entire deltoid muscle to the triceps insertion, at least as assessed by MMT.

No patient who has undergone this procedure has complained about loss of preoperative shoulder function or strength. Furthermore, there has been a tendency in recent years to harvest the posterior half of the muscle rather than the posterior third only, as initially advocated by Moberg.

In the absence of the distal head of the pectoralis major, Allieu and colleagues [19] has stressed the risk of loss of anterior stability of the shoulder after transfer of the posterior deltoid to the triceps. In such a case, he advocates either a change of indications to a biceps transfer or a previous surgical step rebalancing the shoulder by transfer of the anterior head of the deltoid more medially on the clavicle, as described by Buntine and Johnstone [20].

Incomplete passive elbow extension is frequently seen among tetraplegic patients, commonly as a consequence of the unopposed pull of the biceps and other elbow flexors. In the authors' experience, if the elbow can be passively extended to within 30 degrees of full extension, the patient is a potential candidate for deltoid to triceps transfer. This amount of contracture can usually be stretched to nearly full extension in the postoperative period.

A fixed extension contracture between 30 and 45 degrees should be managed by either exercise or surgery as a separate procedure. Once nearly full passive extension has been achieved and the patient has regained strong elbow flexion, one can proceed to deltoid to triceps transfer. For patients in whom the elbow flexion contracture exceeds 45 degrees, the authors prefer to perform biceps to triceps transfer. The greater the flexion contracture, the more likely is the recommendation for biceps to triceps transfer. In this case, the biceps is usually a deforming force contributing to the flexion contracture at the elbow and keeping the forearm in a supinated posture. This deforming force should be treated by tendon lengthening or tenotomy. Rather than lengthening the biceps tendon, which always weakens this muscle, the authors prefer to transfer it.

Comparison with outcome of biceps to triceps transfer

The authors' results of biceps to triceps transfer are not as impressive as that of deltoid to triceps transfer. This difference is most likely a consequence of patient selection. All biceps to triceps cases performed by the authors have been in the circumstances of a significant fixed preoperative elbow flexion contracture, usually exceeding

45 degrees and often requiring anterior capsular release and tendon lengthening of the contracted brachialis muscle, or a weak deltoid muscle, indicating a higher level of spinal cord injury.

Typically, patients cannot actively extend through a large range against the force of gravity; however, these patients do appreciate a gain in the ability to position the arm more accurately in space.

One might anticipate that the transfer of an antagonist may cause problems in rehabilitating the transfer. One of the authors' patients had a less than satisfactory outcome because of durable co-contractions of the brachialis during attempted elbow extension.

Most published series report some loss of elbow flexion strength [15,20,21]. In a report of his experience with 13 elbows in eight patients, Revol [22] stated that flexion torque decreased by a mean of 47% following transfer. Nevertheless, no patient complained about this loss of flexion power, and no activities of daily living were impaired.

Part two: biceps to triceps transfer

Restoration of elbow extension is an integral part of upper extremity surgical reconstruction in persons with tetraplegia. Active elbow extension results in functional gains, including increasing available workspace, performing pressure relief maneuvers, propelling a manual wheelchair, enhancing self-care and leisure activities, operating a vehicle, and promoting independent transfer [22–34]. Elbow extension is considered fundamental toward achieving greater independence. Elbow extension against gravity further enhances these activities, achieving activity above the shoulder level and enhancing reachable workspace (Fig. 11) [4]. Strong elbow extension is also a requirement for upper extremity ambulation using crutches or other support mechanisms.

Posterior deltoid to triceps and biceps to triceps transfers are useful methods to restore active elbow extension [22–34]. The authors previously compared these two techniques in a prospective randomized study [33]. All arms were followed up prospectively for at least 2 years after surgery. Elbow extension was restored in eight arms via the deltoid and in eight arms via the biceps. At 24 months' follow-up, seven of the eight biceps transfers produced antigravity strength (grade 3 or better). In contrast, only one arm with the deltoid transfer was able to extend against gravity. Since that study, we have

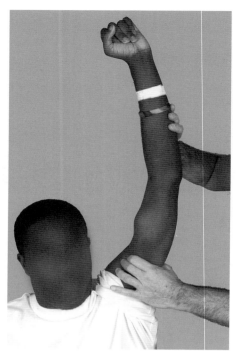

Fig. 11. Full antigravity elbow extension after biceps to triceps tendon transfer achieves activity above the shoulder level and enhances reachable workspace. (*Courtesy of* Shriners Hospital for Children, Philadelphia, PA; with permission.)

exclusively performed biceps to triceps transfer. This article provides an update of our results of biceps to triceps transfers with regards to operative indications, surgical technique, rehabilitation, and outcome.

Operative indications

Active brachialis and supinator muscles are prerequisites for biceps transfer to maintain elbow flexion and forearm supination [28,31,33,35]. The evaluation of their integrity requires a careful physical examination of elbow flexion and forearm supination strength. The brachialis and supinator muscles can be palpated independently of the biceps muscle. Effortless forearm supination without resistance induces supinator function that can be palpated along the proximal radius. Similarly, powerless elbow flexion incites palpable brachialis contraction along the anterior humerus. Equivocal cases require additional evaluation to ensure adequate supinator and brachialis muscle activity [28,31,36]. The authors prefer injection of the biceps muscle with a local anesthetic (eg,

bupivacaine) to induce temporary paralysis of the biceps, which allows an independent assessment of brachialis and supinator function.

A supple elbow with near complete range of motion is also required [30,37]. Patients with an elbow contracture require therapy to resolve the contracture before surgery. Numerous modalities can correct the contracture, although serial casting is the most efficacious method for the authors. Surgery is delayed until the contracture is less than 20 degrees. A greater contracture prevents the biceps tendon from reaching the olecranon at the time of surgery.

Surgical technique

The biceps tendon is routed around the medial side of the humerus [28,30,31,36]. The medial method routes the biceps tendon over the ulnar nerve, which is nonfunctional in persons with tetraplegia who require restoration of elbow extension. A 3-cm anterior transverse incision across the antecubital fossa is performed. The incision can be extended in an L-shaped fashion toward the radial tuberosity to increase the exposure. The musculocutaneous nerve is identified just lateral to the biceps tendon and is protected throughout the procedure. The lacertus fibrosis is incised adjacent to the biceps tendon with protection of the underlying median nerve and brachial artery. The biceps tendon is traced into the forearm toward its insertion into the radial tuberosity. Crossing cubital veins must be ligated. Elbow flexion and forearm supination facilitate identification of the radial tuberosity. Under direct visualization, the biceps tendon is released from the tuberosity, and a large nonabsorbable polyester braided grasping suture is placed within the tendon (Fig. 12). The biceps tendon and muscle are freed from their surrounding attachments within the arm to enhance excursion and improve their line of pull. A second 5- to 7-cm longitudinal incision is made along the medial intermuscular septum. Through the medial incision, the medial intermuscular incision is released and the ulnar nerve identified.

A third 5- to 7-cm posterior incision is made over the distal third of the triceps. The triceps is sharply split over the tip of the olecranon (Fig. 13). Previously, a suture tied over a bony bridge was used to secure the biceps tendon within the olecranon. More recently, a bioabsorbable tenodesis screw (Arthrex, Naples, Florida) is used to secure the biceps tendon within the olecranon. The size of the tendon is measured and

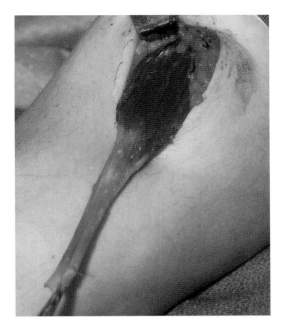

Fig. 12. The biceps tendon is released from the tuberosity and freed from its surrounding attachments within the arm to enhance excursion and improve its line of pull. (*Courtesy of* Shriners Hospital for Children, Philadelphia, PA; with permission.)

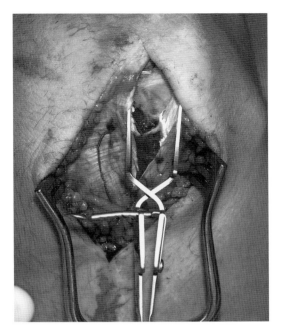

Fig. 13. The distal aspect of the triceps is sharply split over the tip of the olecranon. (*Courtesy of* Shriners Hospital for Children, Philadelphia, PA; with permission.)

a similar size tenodesis screw selected (Fig. 14). A cannulated system is used to prepare the ulna. A drill is passed from the tip of the olecranon into the shaft of the ulna. A cannulated reamer, 1-cm larger than the tendon, is passed over the drill to enlarge the hole.

The biceps tendon is passed from the anterior incision to the medial incision (Fig. 15). The tendon is then directed superficial to the ulnar nerve into the posterior incision. The biceps tendon is subsequently passed obliquely through the medial portion of the triceps tendon using a tendon braider and into the split within the triceps tendon (Fig. 16). The tendon is secured within the olecranon using the tenodesis screw to obtain firm fixation (Fig. 17). This maneuver automatically sets the tension within the tendon transfer. Additional sutures are added between the biceps and triceps tendon.

The limb is maintained in full extension and the subcutaneous tissue and skin closed with nonabsorbable sutures. The tourniquet is deflated, and a well-padded, long-arm cast is applied in the operating room. The wrist is included within the cast; the hand position depends upon concomitant

procedures performed for hand function. The cast is split before leaving the operation room.

Rehabilitation

After surgery, the elbow is placed in a cast in full extension for 3 to 4 weeks. An elbow

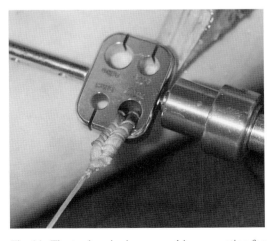

Fig. 14. The tendon size is measured in preparation for tenodesis screw selection. (*Courtesy of* Shriners Hospital for Children, Philadelphia, PA; with permission.)

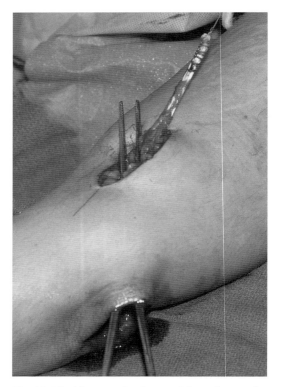

Fig. 15. The biceps tendon is passed from the anterior incision to the medial incision. (*Courtesy of* Shriners Hospital for Children, Philadelphia, PA; with permission.)

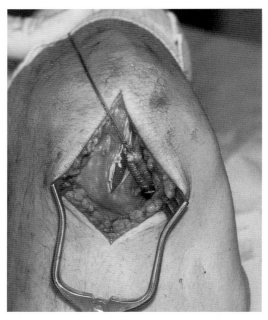

Fig. 16. Biceps tendon in the posterior incision adjacent to split in triceps tendon. (*Courtesy of* Shriners Hospital for Children, Philadelphia, PA; with permission.)

extension splint in full extension is then fabricated for nighttime use. A dial-hinge brace (eg, Bledsoe Brace Systems, Prairie, Texas) is fitted for daytime use and begins as a flexion block at 15 degrees (Fig. 18). The brace is adjusted each week to allow an additional 15 degrees of flexion. The brace is not advanced if an extension lag develops. Tendon transfer firing is started in an antigravity plane. The medially routed biceps can be palpated along the medial humerus during active elbow extension. Verbal prompting of active elbow flexion and active forearm supination facilitate motor learning.

Functional activities of daily living are incorporated into the therapy as elbow flexion increases each week. A dial-hinge brace is continued until 90 degrees of elbow flexion is obtained without an extension lag. A nighttime extension splint is maintained until 12 weeks after surgery. Strengthening is started 3 months after surgery. Occasionally, difficulties are encountered in performing active isolated elbow flexion or extension

movements even though there is clinical evidence of palpable muscle activation within the elbow flexors (brachioradialis and brachialis) or transferred elbow extensor (biceps). In these cases, surface applied electromyography (EMG) using the Pathway MR-20 Dual Channel EMG System (EMPI, Dallas, Texas) is incorporated into the rehabilitation paradigm to address coactivation issues.

Outcome
Clinical. The authors recently reviewed their last 29 patients (42 arms) who underwent biceps to triceps transfer [38]. Two patients were lost to follow-up; therefore, a total of 27 patients (42 arms) were included in the study cohort. The average age was 17.4 years (range, 11.1–20.7 years). Various concomitant procedures were performed for restoration of hand function.

MMT was performed according to accepted standards [39,40]. Unwanted substitution patterns, such as shoulder external rotation with attempted elbow extension, were prevented. In patients who demonstrated full active movement with gravity-minimized and incomplete motion against gravity (ie, extensor lag), an MMT grade of 3-/5 was assigned. When the patient was able to move through the entire arc against gravity, resistance was

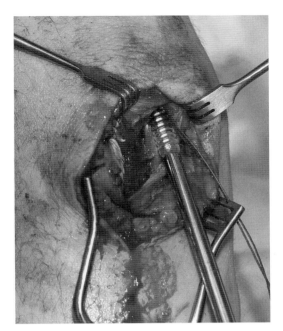

Fig. 17. Biceps tendon secured within the olecranon using the biotenodesis screw. (*Courtesy of* Shriners Hospital for Children, Philadelphia, PA; with permission.)

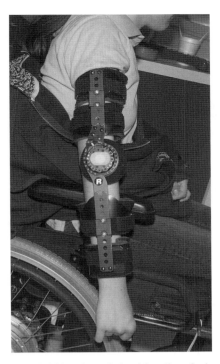

Fig. 18. A dial-hinge brace is fitted for elbow flexion and extension with an advancing flexion block. (*Courtesy of* Shriners Hospital for Children, Philadelphia, PA; with permission.)

imparted against gravity and the muscle strength regraded [39]. A grade 3 MMT implies full motion against gravity without an extensor lag but without the ability to extend the elbow against resistance throughout the arc. A grade 4 MMT indicates the ability of the patient to exert moderate resistance throughout the entire available arc of passive movement. This strict grading criterion eliminates confusion regard the results of MMT and prohibits a patient from being scored grade 4 strength unless they have achieved full available motion against gravity (grade 3 strength).

All patients regained full elbow flexion and forearm supination against gravity and the ability to impart resistance to MMT (grade 4 or 5). No patient expressed subjective complaints of decreased elbow flexion or forearm supination strength (Fig. 19). The average preoperative elbow extension strength was 0.36 (range, 0–1). Stringent MMT for elbow extension revealed an average muscle strength of 3.1 (range, 0–4) (Fig. 20). Thirty-two arms (76%) were able to extend completely against gravity (MMT 3 or greater). Ten arms (24%) were unable to extend completely against gravity (MMT <3), and in six arms the extension problems were directly related to complications. Most patients with less than grade

3 strength were able to impart resistance through some arc against gravity.

Complications occurred from the surgery and during the rehabilitation process. One patient developed a postoperative infection that required irrigation, debridement, and intravenous antibiotics. His follow-up MMT grade was 3-/5. One patient developed an unrecognized compartment syndrome that resulted in denervation of the transfer and a grade 0/5 manual muscle score.

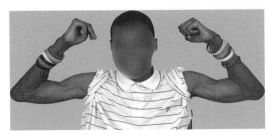

Fig. 19. Full strong elbow flexion following bilateral biceps to triceps tendon transfers. (*Courtesy of* Shriners Hospital for Children, Philadelphia, PA; with permission.)

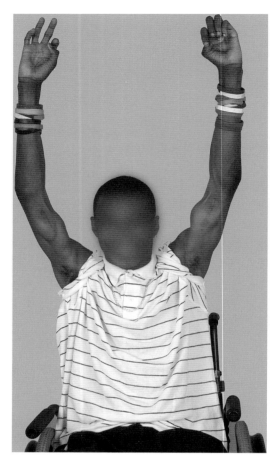

Fig. 20. Grade 4/5 elbow extension following bilateral biceps to triceps tendon transfers. (*Courtesy of* Shriners Hospital for Children, Philadelphia, PA; with permission.)

Four patients attenuated their transfer during rehabilitation. All of these patients had their biceps tendon secured within the olecranon using a suture tied over a bony bridge Three patients have undergone revision and re-attachment of the biceps to the olecranon.

Dynamic EMG analysis. The authors have also reported the dynamic EMG findings after biceps to triceps tendon transfer [41]. Seven subjects (12 arms) averaging 22 ($\pm$0.69) months after biceps to triceps tendon transfer were available for dynamic EMG analysis and MMT. EMG data were synchronized with the electrogoniometric data during (1) a single elbow extension and a single elbow flexion movement, (2) alternating elbow extension and flexion movements at a comfortable

speed, and (3) isometric elbow extension and isometric elbow flexion.

The EMG results provide convincing evidence that the biceps EMG phasic activity changed from an elbow flexor to extensor following transfer. Furthermore, the brachioradialis retained its elbow flexor activity despite being transferred for wrist extension or pinch (Fig. 21). These findings were consistent for both static (isometric) and dynamic (single and alternating) conditions.

Discussion

Upper extremity restoration after spinal cord injury is paramount to independence, dressing, and wheelchair mobility. In a survey of adult men with tetraplegia, most preferred restoration of hand function before bowel, bladder, or sexual function, or walking ability [42]. Because the triceps muscle (C7) is usually paralyzed after tetraplegia, the surgical plan includes restoration of elbow extension [23,25,28,31,33,43]. Active elbow extension results in functional gains and provides an antagonist to elbow flexion that counteracts the flexion moment produced after brachioradialis tendon transfer [28,34].

Early reports of biceps to triceps tendon transfer used either a medial or lateral routing technique [24,27,31,35,43,44]. Friedenberg [27] in 1954 initially described the lateral method and reported on two bilateral cases. Ejeskar [24] reported on the lateral route in 1988 in five patients and noted the first complication of radial nerve palsy, which resulted in a degradation of hand function. The medial route for biceps to triceps tendon transfer avoids the radial nerve [28,30,31,33,35]. Kuz and colleagues [31] reported on the technique of medial routing and the outcome in three patients (four cases). All of the patients achieved at least grade 4 elbow

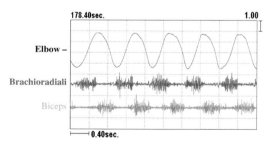

Fig. 21. EMG following biceps to triceps transfer demonstrating phasic reversal with the biceps acting as an elbow extensor and the brachioradialis as an elbow flexor.

extension strength without a functional loss of elbow flexion strength. Revol and colleagues [35]
also reported on the medial route for biceps to triceps transfer in eight patients (13 elbows). The
mean postoperative active range of motion was
from 6 degrees of extension to 137 degrees of flexion. Mean elbow flexion power was measured before and after surgery in eight patients. A 47%
reduction was noted, although no patient complained about any functional impact. Functional
integration of the elbow extension was evident in
all patients.

The authors performed a prospective randomized study to evaluate and compare the deltoid to
triceps and biceps to triceps transfers for restoration of elbow extension [33]. Sixteen arms (9 patients) were included and randomly assigned to
undergo a deltoid to triceps transfer or a biceps
to triceps transfer. All of the arms were candidates
for either procedure and were followed up prospectively for at least 2 years after surgery. Elbow
extension was restored in eight arms via the
deltoid and in eight arms via the biceps. At
24 months' follow-up, seven of the eight biceps
transfers produced antigravity strength (grade
3 or better). In contrast, only one arm with the
deltoid transfer was able to extend against gravity.
There was a significant but subclinical loss of
elbow flexion torque following both transfers.
Three months after surgery, the deltoid group
showed a 51% loss of elbow flexion torque and
the biceps group a 52% loss of elbow flexion torque. By 24 months after surgery, both groups
improved but still showed an average loss of
32% for the deltoid group and 47% for the biceps
group. Nevertheless, no subject noted any functional consequences attributed to the loss of elbow
flexion torque. This study changed our treatment
recommendations for surgical reconstruction of
elbow extension. Subsequently, only the biceps
to triceps transfer was recommended for restoration of elbow extension. Since then, we have also
used the biceps to triceps transfer to salvage failed
deltoid to triceps tendon transfers [29].

The strength results of the deltoid to triceps
transfer in our prospective study mirrored our
larger unpublished clinical series. With few exceptions, patients who have undergone the deltoid to
triceps transfer are unable to consistently produce
antigravity strength long term (2 or more years)
after surgery, regardless of the type of interposi-
tion graft used. There are multiple possible causes
of the inferior results, including surgical technique, attenuation of the transfer over time, and

a faulty rehabilitation protocol with inadequate
protection of the transfer [45]. In fact, other
researchers have reported better results of the
deltoid to triceps transfer. Mohammed and colleagues [32] evaluated elbow extension results
after the deltoid to triceps transfer using Moberg's
technique with a tibialis anterior free tendon graft.
Twenty-four transfers were performed, and 71%
achieved against-gravity strength. Lacey and colleagues [14] reported the successful outcomes of
16 posterior deltoid transfers. Median muscle
strength was grade 3 (range, 2–4), and only one
transfer was less than grade 3. Raczka and colleagues [13] reviewed 23 arms in 22 patients. Eigh-
teen arms were available for follow-up an average
of 49 months from surgery. Thirteen arms were
graded as muscle strength 3 or greater. Paul and
colleagues [34] reported on 11 patients who underwent 12 deltoid transfers. Nine patients (10 arms)
were followed up for an average of 31 months.
The average muscle grade was 3.4, with seven of
nine arms obtaining grade 3 strength or better.
None of these studies describe the rigors of the
MMT procedure that we have adopted. Our stringent methodology during MMT lends confidence
to the accuracy and repeatability of the strength
results.

Even with the positive reports of the deltoid
transfer, there are clear advantages of the biceps
transfer with regards to surgical technique, outcome, and rehabilitation. First, the biceps to
triceps transfer is a straightforward procedure
that avoids any intervening graft. Tension is
simple to set via direct insertion on the bicep's
tendon into the olecranon. Second, the biceps to
triceps transfer uniformly produces antigravity
strength as an expected outcome. Our cohort
was able to achieve full antigravity strength 76%
of the time. Of the ten arms that were unable to
extend completely against gravity (MMT <3), the
results in six arms were directly related to complications. Lastly, the deltoid to triceps transfer
has demanding postoperative restrictions when
compared with the biceps to triceps transfer. The
lesser limitations of biceps to triceps transfer are
especially important for impaired persons with
tetraplegia [30,31,35].

In the authors' experience, the outcome of
elbow extension has substantially improved since
changing from a deltoid to triceps transfer to
a biceps to triceps transfer. The latter cohort of
patients supports our clinical impression that the
biceps to triceps transfer should be the preferred
technique for elbow extension in persons with

tetraplegia. Furthermore, EMG study shows that
the biceps can be trained to activate preferentially
during elbow extension, a reversal of its ordinary
action as an elbow flexor. There are critical
prerequisites to ensure a satisfactory outcome.
These factors include intact brachialis and supinator muscles, resolution of any elbow contracture, and careful postoperative rehabilitation.
Failure to adhere to these prerequisites, such as
broadening the indications to contracted limbs
with fixed deformities or spastic limbs, will
directly diminish the outcome [10,24].

Summary

Reconstruction of elbow extension, whether
using a deltoid to triceps or biceps to triceps
transfer, has been the single most satisfying
reconstruction for the authors' patients. Even
though the overall time for rehabilitation can
be relatively lengthy, the functional gain is substantial, predictable, and easily appreciated by
the patient. Furthermore, the risks to residual
preoperative function are practically nil. The
transfer procedure represents an important
addition to our reconstructive surgical
armamentarium.

References

[1] Merle d'Aubigne M, Seddon H, Hendy A, et al.
Tendons transfers. Proceedings of the Royal Society
of Medicine 1949;48:831–7.
[2] Moberg E. Surgical treatment for absent single-hand
grip and elbow extension in quadriplegia: principles
and preliminary experience. J Bone Joint Surg Am
1975;57(2):196–206.
[3] Allieu Y, Teissier J, Triki F, et al. Restoration of elbow extension in the tetraplegic by transplantation
of the posterior deltoid: study of 21 cases). Rev
Chir Orthop Reparatrice Appar Mot 1985;71(3):
195–200 [in French].
[4] Lacey SH, Wilber RG, Peckham PH, et al. The posterior deltoid to triceps transfer: a clinical and biomechanical assessment. J Hand Surg [Am] 1986;
11(4):542–7.
[5] Lamb DW. Upper limb surgery in tetraplegia.
J Hand Surg [Br] 1989;14(2):143–4.
[6] Hentz VR, Brown M, Keoshian LA, et al. Upper
limb reconstruction in quadriplegia: functional assessment and proposed treatment modifications. J
Hand Surg [Am] 1983;8(2):119–31.
[7] Castro-Serra A, Lopez-Pita A. A new technique to
correct triceps paralysis. Hand 1983;15:42–6.

[8] Johnstone BR, Jordan CJ, Buntine JA, et al. A review of surgical rehabilitation of the upper limb in
quadriplegia. Paraplegia 1988;26(5):317–39.
[9] Mennen U, Boonzaier AC. An improved technique
of posterior deltoid to triceps transfer in tetraplegia.
J Hand Surg [Br] 1991;16(2):197–201.
[10] Moberg E. Surgical rehabilitation of the upper limb
in tetraplegia. Paraplegia 1990;28(5):330–4.
[11] Bryan RS. The Moberg deltoid-triceps replacement
and key-pinch operations in quadriplegia: preliminary experiences. Hand 1977;9(3):207–14.
[12] DeBenedetti M. Restoration of elbow extension
power in the tetraplegic patient using the Moberg
technique. J Hand Surg [Am] 1979;4(1):86–9.
[13] Raczka R, Braun R, Waters RL, et al. Posterior deltoid-to-triceps transfer in quadriplegia. Clin Orthop
Relat Res 1984;(187):163–7.
[14] Rabischong E, Benoit P, Benichou M, et al. Length-
tension relationship of the posterior deltoid to
triceps transfer in C6 tetraplegic patients. Paraplegia
1993;31:33–9.
[15] Ejeskar A, Dahllof A. Results of reconstructive
surgery in the upper limb of tetraplegic patients.
Paraplegia 1988;26(3):204–8.
[16] Lieber RL, Fridén J, Hobbs T, et al. Analysis of
posterior deltoid function one year after surgical
restoration of elbow extension. J Hand Surg [Am]
2003;28(2):288–93.
[17] Hentz VR, Leclercq C. Surgical rehabilitation of the
upper limb in tetraplegia. London: Saunders; 2002.
p. 97–118.
[18] Moberg E. The upper limb in tetraplegia: a new
approach to surgical rehabilitation. Stuttgart
(Germany): George Thieme; 1978.
[19] Allieu Y, Benichou M, Ohanna F, et al. [Func-
tional surgery of the upper limbs in tetraplegic
patients: current trends after 10 years of
experience at the Propara Center]. Rev Chir
Orthop Reparatrice Appar Mot 1993;79(2):79–88
[in French].
[20] Buntine JA, Johnstone BR. The contributions of
plastic surgery to care of the spinal cord injured
patient. Paraplegia 1988;26(2):87–93.
[21] Zancolli E, Zancolli E Jr. Tetraplégies traumatiques.
In: Tubiana R, editor. Traité de Chirurgie de la
Main. Paris: Masson; 1991.
[22] Beasley R. Surgical treatment of hands for C5-C6
tetraplegia. Orthop Clin North Am 1983;14:
893–904.
[23] Dunkerley AL, Ashburn A, Stack EL. Deltoid
triceps transfer and functional independence of
people with tetraplegia. Spinal Cord 2000;38:
435–41.
[24] Ejeskär A. Upper limb surgical rehabilitation in
high-level tetraplegia. Hand Clin 1988;585–99.
[25] Falconer DP. Tendon transfers about the shoulder
and elbow in the spinal cord injured patient. Hand
Clin 1988;4(2):211–21.

[26] Freehafer AA, Kelly CM, Peckham PH. Tendon transfer for the restoration of upper limb function after a cervical spinal cord injury. J Hand Surg 1984;9A:887–93.

[27] Friedenberg ZB. Transposition of the biceps brachii for triceps weakness. J Bone Joint Surg 1954;36A: 656–8.

[28] Kozin SH. Tetraplegia. Journal of the American Society for Surgery of the Hand 2002;3:141–52.

[29] Kozin SH, Schloth C. Bilateral biceps-to-triceps transfer to salvage bilateral deltoid-to-triceps transfer: a case report. J Hand Surg [Am] 2002;27: 666–9.

[30] Kozin SH. Biceps-to-triceps transfer for restoration of elbow extension in tetraplegia. Techniques in Hand and Upper Extremity Surgery 2003;7:43–51.

[31] Kuz J, Van Heest AE, House JH. Biceps-to-triceps transfer in tetraplegic patients: report of the medial routing technique and follow-up of three cases. J Hand Surg 1999;24A:161–72.

[32] Mohammand K, Rothwell A, Sinclair S, et al. Upper limb surgery for tetraplegia. J Bone Joint Surg 1992; 74B:873–9.

[33] Mulcahey MJ, Lutz C, Kozin SH, et al. Prospective evaluation of biceps to triceps and deltoid to triceps for elbow extension in tetraplegia. J Hand Surg [Am] 2003;28:964–71.

[34] Paul SD, Gellman H, Waters P, et al. Single-stage reconstruction of key pinch and extension of the elbow in tetraplegic patients. J Bone Joint Surg 1994; 76A:1451–6.

[35] Revol M, Briand E, Servant JM, et al. Biceps-to-triceps transfer in tetraplegia: the medial route. J Hand Surg [Br] 1999;24(2):235–7.

[36] McDowell CL, Moberg EA, House JH. The second international conference on surgical rehabilitation of the upper limb in tetraplegia (quadriplegia). J Hand Surg 1986;11A:604–8.

[37] Hentz VR, Hamlin C, Keoshian L. Surgical reconstruction in tetraplegia. Hand Clin 1988;4:601–7.

[38] Kozin SH, D'Addesi L, Duffy T, et al. Biceps to triceps transfer for elbow extension in persons with tetraplegia. Presented at the 61st Annual Meeting, American Society for Surgery of the Hand, Washington, DC, September 2006.

[39] Clarkson HM, Gilewich GB. Musculoskeletal assessment: joint range of motion and manual muscle strength. Baltimore (MD): Williams & Wilkins; 1988. p. 20–6.

[40] Hislop H. Daniels and Worthingham's muscle testing: techniques of manual examination. Philadelphia: W.B. Saunders; 2002.

[41] Hutchinson D, Kozin SH, Mulcahey MJ, et al. Dynamic EMG changes in the biceps following transfer for elbow extension in persons with tetraplegia. Dallas (TX): American Spinal Injury Association; 2005.

[42] Hanson RW, Franklin MR. Sexual loss in relation to other functional losses for spinal cord injured males. Arch Phys Med Rehabil 1976;57:291–3.

[43] Zancolli E. Functional restoration of the upper limbs in traumatic quadriplegia. In: Zancolli E, editor. Structural and dynamic bases of hand surgery. 2nd edition. Philadelphia: Lippincott; 1979. p. 229–62.

[44] Zancolli EA. Tetraplegia. In: McFarlane RM, editor. Unsatisfactory results in hand surgery: the hand and upper limb. New York: Churchill Livingstone; 1987. p. 274–80.

[45] Friden J, Lieber RL. Quantitative evaluation of the posterior deltoid to triceps tendon transfer based on muscle architectural properties. J Hand Surg [Am] 2001;26:147–55.

ELSEVIER
SAUNDERS

Hand Clin 24 (2008) 203–213

HAND
CLINICS

Pediatric Onset Spinal Cord Injury: Implications on Management of the Upper Limb in Tetraplegia

Scott H. Kozin, MD[a,b,*]

[a]*Department of Orthopaedic Surgery, Temple University 3401 North Broad Street, Philadelphia, PA 19140, USA*
[b]*Pediatric Hand and Upper Extremity Center of Excellence, Shriners Hospitals for Children,
3551 North Broad Street, Philadelphia, PA 19140, USA*

Spinal cord injury (SCI) most frequently occurs in persons between 16 and 30 years of age. In the United States, motor vehicle crashes and violence are the primary causes of SCI. Violence is a more common cause of injury among individuals who are younger, male, or African American [1–3]. Pediatric SCI is less common and has some particular features unique to children. Boys outnumber girls by a ratio of approximately 4:1 in adolescent and childhood SCI; however, the frequency of SCI in boys and girls under 5 years of age is similar. In addition, the mechanism of injury is often different in children. Unique pediatric mechanisms include birth trauma, falls, child abuse, tumor, and infection (eg, transverse myelitis) (Fig. 1) [4–9]. In addition, children with skeletal dysplasias, juvenile rheumatoid arthritis, and Down syndrome are predisposed to cervical SCI [10].

Younger children are also prone to sustain an SCI without radiographic abnormality (SCIWORA) when compared with older adolescents or adults. Approximately 60% of children who sustain an SCI at 10 years of age or younger will have SCIWORA, in contrast to 20% of older children and adolescents [11]. Despite the benign radiologic picture of SCIWORA, these children are more likely to have complete lesions [11]. Another unique feature of pediatric onset SCI is a delay of 30 minutes to 4 days in the onset of

neurologic abnormalities in about 25% to 50% of children who sustain a SCI [1]. Children with delayed onset of neurologic findings may initially experience transient and subtle neurologic symptoms, such as paresthesias or subjective weakness.

The life expectancy for children and adolescents with SCI is somewhat less than that for the general population and is a function of neurologic level and category [1,3]. The less severe the SCI in respect to level and completeness, the longer the expected survival. Children who have SCI have similar expectations of medicine and rehabilitation as their adult peers. Children and youth who have SCI return to school and are expected to engage in activities associated with school and home chores [2]. In these roles, they need to reach up to write on chalkboards and are expected to support their bodies during transfers in and out of the wheelchair. Children who have SCI participate in typical age-defined clubs, such as Boy Scouts, Girl Scouts, choirs, and youth programs. The role of the upper extremity is pivotal in their lives. This article focuses on the pediatric upper limb after SCI and highlights the obstacles during reconstruction.

Initial evaluation

At the author's center, we focus on pediatric SCI and act as a regional and national referral center. We use a comprehensive multidisciplinary team approach with input from a variety of specialties, including nurses, therapists, physiatrists, spine surgeons, and upper extremity surgeons. A global treatment plan is formulated

---
* Pediatric Hand and Upper Extremity Center of Excellence, Shriners Hospitals for Children, 3551 North Broad Street, Philadelphia, PA 19140.
E-mail address: skozin@shrinenet.org

0749-0712/08/$ - see front matter © 2008 Elsevier Inc. All rights reserved.
doi:10.1016/j.hcl.2008.02.004

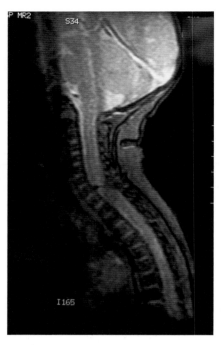

Fig. 1. MRI of a 4-year-old boy who had SCI during the birthing process. (*Courtesy of* Shriners Hospital for Children, Philadelphia, PA; with permission.)

addressing the various needs of the child from skin care through locomotion. If upper extremity surgery is being contemplated, the input from the team is critical in the decision-making process; therefore, the initial admission usually requires a few days to allow a complete assessment by all services.

The initial evaluation of a child requires patience, empathy, knowledge, and a support staff. The rapport between doctor and family should be in lay terms with avoidance of medical jargon. Misconceptions concerning SCI are common and should be dispelled. The concept of a "cure" is always in their minds, and the team should be prepared to answer. Parents often feel some guilt about the SCI, and these feelings should be recognized and addressed. Children with SCI require medical, psychologic, financial, and social assistance. This type of care is best provided at an institution familiar with the care of children with SCI, and referral is warranted.

Preoperative considerations

The preoperative evaluation is similar in children and adolescents. The examination of a child is always challenging. The evaluation of a child who

has SCI is even more difficult. Age-appropriate instructions and testing is crucial. The assessment of manual muscle testing is even more difficult in young children because effort is hard to elicit.

Age at surgery

The exact age for surgery after pediatric SCI is unknown, and guidelines are unavailable. We assess the child from a physical, neurologic, emotional, and maturity standpoint. Nerve recovery should plateau before upper extremity reconstruction; however, the doctrine of waiting 18 months after injury does not appear to be justified in complete SCI. Complete injury often recovers a spinal cord level of function within the first 3 to 6 months after spinal column stabilization. After this time, the chances of regaining nerve and muscle activity that will alter function are negligible; therefore, upper extremity reconstruction may be contemplated after complete SCI without any considerable change in neurologic status over the previous 3 months. This early reconstruction concept fosters sooner independence, better ability to perform activities of daily living, and quicker reintroduction into society. This principle of early intervention does not apply to incomplete SCI. Such injury is less predictable regarding recovery, usually asymmetric, and often has a considerable spastic component; therefore, it is more difficult to formulate a reconstruction plan.

Crucial items to consider are the ability of the child to participate in the postoperative regimen and the availability of family support. In complete SCI, the planned procedure is unlikely to change over time; however, the maturity level of the child is likely to improve. If the therapist believes that the child can and will not cooperate after surgery, the surgery is delayed until the child is older. The evaluation must consider the pros and cons of surgery, and rhetoric is necessary between the surgeon and therapist. Successful surgery will improve independence, whereas unsuccessful surgery may further impair upper extremity function. Furthermore, secondary surgery for tendon rupture or adhesions is difficult and the results mediocre; therefore, the timing of surgery is a critical decision and requires substantial consideration. In general, we are unlikely to operate on a child before school age but will perform surgery during elementary school.

Assessment

The upper extremities of children who have tetraplegia have similar features as adult onset SCI with a few notable exceptions [12]. The upper extremity examination should be detailed with an assessment and documentation of active range of motion and passive range of motion of the entire upper extremity. If possible, pinch and grip strength measurements should be recorded. A modified device may be necessary to accommodate the small hand and the weak force production. In addition, examination should include an observation of prehensile patterns and adaptive maneuvers. Children are notorious at figuring out ways to accomplish desirable tasks, and these "adaptations" need to be recognized and the effect of surgery considered. For example, children without pinch or grasp will write while holding the pen with two hands, and surgery for pinch may change this prehensile pattern. This adjustment needs to be recognized before surgery so that the child and parent understand the goal is unilateral penmanship and an adjustment in writing pattern (Fig. 2).

Manual muscle testing is a subjective and objective evaluation of muscle strength. Manual muscle testing is performed according to accepted standards [13,14]. Unwanted substitution patterns, such as shoulder external rotation with attempted elbow extension, are prevented. An additional confounding factor in grading muscle strength is the questionable ability of a child to cooperate during resistance testing.

The examination should classify the child according to the American Spinal Injury Association

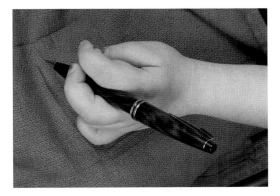

Fig. 2. Photograph of a 10-year-old following pinch and grasp reconstruction who has a change in the prehensile pattern and the ability to write with one hand. (*Courtesy of* Shriners Hospital for Children, Philadelphia, PA; with permission.)

(ASIA) or the International Classification of Surgery of the Hand in Tetraplegia (ICSHT), devised at the First International Conference on Surgical Rehabilitation of the Upper Limb in Tetraplegia in 1984 (Table 1) [15]. In contrast to the ASIA system, the ICSHT is designed to guide surgical reconstruction of the upper limb in tetraplegia (Table 2). The system categorizes patients by the number of muscles below the elbow with grade 4 manual muscle strength or greater. This scheme is critical to understand and provides an inventory of muscles available for transfer and guidelines for surgical management.

The classification also characterizes limb sensibility as cutaneous (Cu) or ocular (O). Intact cutaneous sensibility implies two-point

Table 1
International Classification of Surgery of the Hand in Tetraplegia

Sensibility	Group	Muscle	Function
Cutaneous (Cu) or ocular (O)	0	No muscles below elbow suitable for transfer	
	1	Brachioradialis	Flexion of elbow
	2	Extensor carpi radialis longus	Weak wrist extension with radial deviation
	3	Extensor carpi radialis brevis	Wrist extension
	4	Pronator teres	Forearm pronation
	5	Flexor carpi radialis	Wrist flexion
	6	Extensor digitorum communis	Finger metacarpophalangeal joint extension (extrinsic extension of the fingers)
	7	Extensor pollicis longus	Thumb interphalangeal joint extension (extrinsic extension of the thumb)
	8	Digital flexors	Extrinsic finger flexion
	9	All muscles except intrinsics	
	X	Exceptions	

Table 2

Surgical guidelines based on the International Classification of Surgery of the Hand in Tetraplegia

Group	Recommended procedure	Alternatives
0	Functional electrical stimulation	
1	BR → ECRB, FPL tenodesis, FPL split tenodesis, ± EPL tenodesis, ± thumb CMC fusion	Functional electrical stimulation
2	Same as 1 except BR →FPL instead of FPL tenodesis, ± thumb CMC fusion	Functional electrical stimulation
3	Same as 2 plus ECRL→FDP	Stage I: extensor & intrinsic tenodesis, FPL split tenodesis, ± thumb CMC fusion Stage II: BR →FPL, ECRL→FDP
4	Same as 3 or BR → EDC & EPL, PT → FPL, FPL split tenodesis, intrinsic tenodesis, ECRL→FDP (needs 2 stages)	PT → EDC & EPL, BR → FPL, FPL split tenodesis, intrinsic tenodesis, ECRL→FDP (needs 2 stages)
5	Same as 4	Same as 4
6	BR → FPL; FPL split tenodesis, EPL → EDC, intrinsic tenodesis, ECRL→FDP, ± thumb CMC fusion	
7	Same as 6 except no EPL → EDC	
8	BR→FPL, active intrinsic transfer	ECRL → FDS
9	Active intrinsic transfer	

Abbreviations: BR, brachioradialis; CMC, carpal metacarpal; ECRB, extensor carpi radialis brevis; ECRL, extensor carpi radialis longus; EDC, extensor digitorum communis; EPL, extensor pollicis longus; FDP, flexor digitorum profundus; FDS, flexor digitorum superficialis; FPL, flexor pollicis longus; PT, pronator teres.

discrimination of 10 mm or less within the thumb and index pulp, which is necessary for lateral pinch without eyesight. Ocular sensibility indicates vision as the only afferent; however, sensory examination in the child is complicated. Threshold and functional two-point discrimination are unreliable until about 9 years of age. The wrinkle test is helpful because a positive test indicates some nerve innervation.

Surgical approach

The surgical plan for children follows the adult reconstructive ladder for SCI reconstruction (Table 3). The reconstructive ladder requires a basic understanding of kinematics and normal hand function. Successful manipulation of objects requires acquisition, grasp, manipulation, and release. A combination of extrinsic and intrinsic function leads to a coordinated grasp pattern. This pattern of synchronous grasp and release is markedly disrupted after SCI because the extrinsic muscles, intrinsic muscles, or both are affected.

The reconstruction ladder begins at the first rung, and wrist extension is the prime motion. Wrist extension is the fundamental motion for hand function [16]. Active wrist extension and

subsequent gravity-assisted wrist flexion provide passive tenodesis and marginal hand function. This motion couples wrist extension with digital flexion and wrist flexion with digital extension. Patients without wrist extension (ICSHT groups 0 and 1) have no means to produce tenodesis and are unable to acquire, grasp, or release objects. Patients with group 0 function do not have a suitable donor muscle for transfer and can

Table 3

Reconstructive ladder for hand function in spinal cord injury

Priority		Preferred technique
1	Wrist extension	BR to ECRB
2	Lateral pinch	BR to FPL
3	Grasp	ECRL to FDP
4	Opening	BR to EDC plus passive intrinsicsplasty
5	Coordinated grasp and opposition	FDS intrinsicsplasty plus ECU opponensplasty

Abbreviations: BR, brachioradialis; ECRB, extensor carpi radialis brevis; ECRL, extensor carpi radialis longus; ECU, extensor carpi ulnaris; EDC, extensor digitorum communis; FDS, flexor digitorum superficialis; FDP, flexor digitorum profundus; FPL, flexor pollicus longus.

achieve hand function only through neuropros-thetic implantation [17,18]. Patients with group 1 function do not have wrist motion but have an available brachioradialis muscle for transfer to the extensor carpi radialis brevis muscle for wrist extension. Grasp and released is performed via te-nodesis, which can be enhanced by an orthotic device.

Pinch restoration is the second rung and next most important hand function (Fig. 3) [19]. For activities of daily living, far more tasks are performed with lateral pinch than grasp. This fact underscores the importance of lateral pinch reconstruction for object manipulation, such as holding a toothbrush, pen, fork, or computer disk. A more sophisticated form of pinch (ie, opposition or pulp-to-pulp pinch) requires an op-posable thumb with good control and sensibility. Thumb opposition is a complicated function with components of palmar abduction, flexion, and pronation. Opposition is often beyond the scope of restorability in tetraplegia, unless the SCI is at a lower level with preservation of extrin-sic function and isolated loss of intrinsic function.

Grasp is the third rung and next priority during hand reconstruction (Fig. 4) [16]. As stated previ-ously, synchronous grasp uses extrinsic and intrin-sic muscle activity and is typically unobtainable in tetraplegia. Extrinsic grasp via a tendon transfer to restore flexor digitorum profundus function is

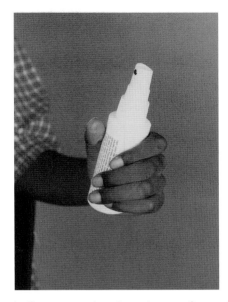

Fig. 4. Grasp restoration via tendon transfer provides the ability to hold objects such as a bottle. (*Courtesy of* Shriners Hospital for Children, Philadelphia, PA; with permission.)

a realistic goal in ICSHT group 3 or greater. This palmar grasp provides the ability to hold ob-jects, although the digital roll-up impedes the ac-quisition of objects with considerable diameter, such as a cup. Persons with tetraplegia compensate for acquisition by using wrist flexion and concom-itant finger extension tenodesis to encircle the item followed by active wrist extension and active finger flexion to maintain the object within the hand.

Finger and thumb extension is the forth rung and next priority in hand reconstruction. This action can often be accomplished by wrist flexion (active or passive) and concomitant passive finger extension tenodesis. Active finger extension is obtainable when sufficient motors exist (ICSHT group 4 or greater). Isolated tender transfer to the extrinsic finger extensors produces metacarpopha-langeal (MCP) joint extension with minimal interphalangeal (IP) joint extension. A passive intrinsic reconstruction to limit MCP joint exten-sion is usually necessary to provide some IP extension. Restoration of both finger flexion and extension requires a two-stage reconstruction because the postoperative rehabilitations are disparate [15]. Furthermore, this concept is ex-tremely difficult to achieve in its entirety. Surgical equilibrium of flexion and extension often results in a slight imbalance toward flexion or extension.

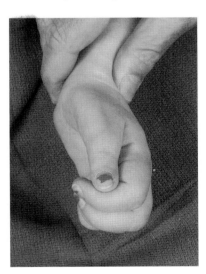

Fig. 3. Lateral pinch restoration via tendon transfer enhances activities of daily living, such as holding a toothbrush, pen, fork, or computer disk. (*Courtesy of* Shriners Hospital for Children, Philadelphia, PA; with permission.)

Intrinsic function is the last priority in hand reconstruction, although some type of passive intrinsic restoration is usually part of finger extension reconstruction. Active intrinsic reconstruction is only indicated in lower level tetraplegia (ICSHT groups 6 or greater) (Fig. 5). In these patients, standard principles and transfers for low median and low ulnar palsies are applicable to recreate coordinated hand function.

Pediatric obstacles and dilemmas

The greatest surgical obstacle is the size of the tendons. Adolescents with SCI have large tendons that make possible tendon transfer with a strong and robust weave. In contrast, young children who are injured have small tendons that are difficult to transfer and weave. An exception to this rule is muscle tendon units that have persistent spasticity following injury, which provides relentless force and promotes muscle-tendon hypertrophy. Unfortunately, these spastic muscle-tendons are usually not appropriate for transfers secondary to lack of volitional control. Various surgical tactics exist to surmount the small size of the tendons, including a reverse weave, suture augmentation, and tendon graft. Usually, the active donor tendon is woven into the recipient tendon using a tendon passer; a reverse weave implies the opposite. For example, standard active pinch transfer requires weaving the brachioradialis through the flexor pollicis longus tendon. In small tendons, the small proximal tendon of the flexor pollicis longus is cut and woven through the larger brachioradialis tendon

(Fig. 6). Regarding suture augmentation, we augment the typical weave with a strong suture material such as Fiberloop (Athrex, Naples, Florida) passed in a running locked fashion across the entire series of tendon weaves. Lastly, an onlay tendon graft (usually the flexor carpi radialis tendon) can be bridged across the coaptation sites and sutured in a running locked fashion. All of these measures enhance the strength of the transfer but do not achieve the rigor of robust adolescent or adult tendon weaves.

Another surgical obstacle in pediatric SCI is the prevalence of fixed contractures secondary to ongoing muscle imbalance since a young age. This imbalance primarily affects the elbow, forearm, and MCP joints. In C5-C6 SCI, the elbow and forearm are prone to develop a contracture. The preponderance of elbow flexors (C5 and C6) and forearm supinators (C5 and C6) combined with the absence of elbow extensors (C7) and forearm pronators (C7 and C8) promotes an elbow flexion and forearm supination posture. Initially, this posture is passively correctable and preventable by therapy and splinting; however, when untreated, a fixed contracture develops over time. We try to resolve these contractures by therapy including modalities such as serial casting, serial static splinting, and dynamic splinting. In elbow contractures that can be resolved, we then consider biceps-to-triceps tendon transfer to augment elbow extension and to rebalance the elbow joint. The technique is similar to that in adults; however, the biceps tendon is not drilled into the olecranon because

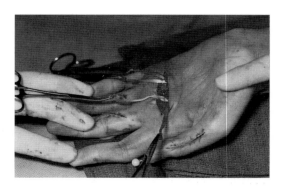

Fig. 5. Intrinsic reconstruction in a child who has lower level tetraplegia using flexor digitorum superficialis intrinsic transfer (ICSHT groups 6 or greater). (*Courtesy of* Shriners Hospital for Children, Philadelphia, PA; with permission.)

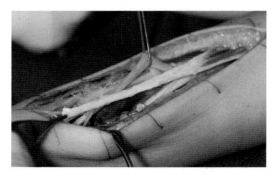

Fig. 6. Active pinch reconstruction via brachioradialis to flexor pollicis longus. Vessel loop around hypoplastic flexor pollicis longus. In this case, the proximal flexor pollicis longus was cut and woven through the larger brachioradialis tendon (ie, reverse weave). (*Courtesy of* Shriners Hospital for Children, Philadelphia, PA; with permission.)

of the open growth plate. Instead, the biceps tendon is woven through the triceps tendon. A prerequisite to biceps-to-triceps transfer is active brachialis and supinator muscles to maintain elbow flexion and forearm supination. Their evaluation requires a careful physical examination of elbow flexion and forearm supination strength. The brachialis and supinator muscles can be palpated independent of the biceps muscle. Effortless forearm supination without resistance induces supinator function that can be palpated along the proximal radius. Similarly, powerless elbow flexion incites palpable brachialis contraction along the anterior humerus. In children, this examination is more difficult. Equivocal cases require additional evaluation to ensure adequate supinator and brachialis muscle activity. We prefer injection of the biceps muscle with a local anesthetic to induce temporary paralysis, which allows independent assessment of brachialis and supinator function.

Failure to correct the contracture to less than 30 degrees requires careful decision making and input from the team. The elbow contracture can be lessened by lengthening of the elbow flexors, primarily the biceps and the brachialis; however, the impact of diminished elbow flexion power needs to be considered in the decision-making process. In these tight elbows, we have not transferred the biceps tension to the triceps because the foreshortened muscle-tendon unit limits excursion

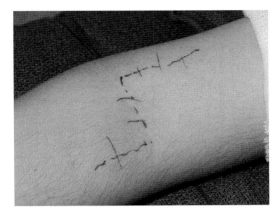

Fig. 8. Six-year-old girl who has supple supination posturing of her left arm secondary to muscle imbalance. Skin incision for biceps rerouting surgery. (*Courtesy of* Shriners Hospital for Children, Philadelphia, PA; with permission.)

and prevents the tendon from reaching the triceps tendon.

The forearm is prone to develop a fixed supination deformity, which complicates reconstruction (Fig. 7). Therapy is the principal modality to regain passive mobility. Restoration of passive forearm rotation allows biceps re-routing to balance the forearm joint (Figs. 8–11). A fixed deformity implies a fixed contracture of the interosseous membrane or an underlying bony deformity [20]. Correction requires a careful assessment of forearm use in activities of daily living, sensibility, and wrist extension. In children with negligible sensibility and lack of wrist extension, the forearm is better positioned in supination. This position allows ocular input to assess objects

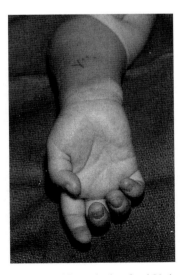

Fig. 7. Eight-year-old boy who has fixed 90-degree supination contracture of his right arm secondary to muscle imbalance. (*Courtesy of* Shriners Hospital for Children, Philadelphia, PA; with permission.)

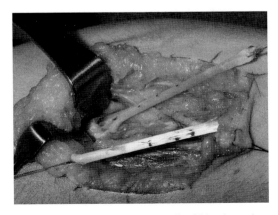

Fig. 9. Z-plasty across entire length of bicep's tendon. (*Courtesy of* Shriners Hospital for Children, Philadelphia, PA; with permission.)

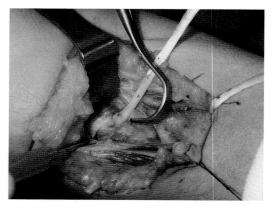

Fig. 10. A curved clamp (Castameda pediatric clamp, Pilling Surgical, Horshan, Pennsylvania) facilitates tendon rerouting around the radius. (*Courtesy of* Shriners Hospital for Children, Philadelphia, PA; with permission.)

within the hand and prevents the wrist from flopping into flexion. In contrast, children with cutaneous sensibility and wrist extension usually benefit from repositioning the forearm into mild pronation. This position promotes active wrist extension and tenodesis prehension.

Surgical methods to reposition the limb include release of the interosseous membrane combined with biceps re-routing, osteotomy of the radius or ulna, and formation of a one-bone forearm [21–23]. We have used all of these methods to correct forearm position. Currently, we favor single bone osteotomy for correction of less than 45 degrees, osteotomies of both bones for correction of up to 90 degrees, and formation of a one-bone

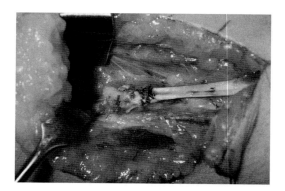

Fig. 11. Tendon passed through interosseous space, around radius, and repaired back to proximal limb using a tendon weave augmented with nonabsorbable suture. (*Courtesy of* Shriners Hospital for Children, Philadelphia, PA; with permission.)

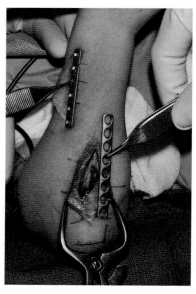

Fig. 12. Osteotomy of the radius and ulna. Fixation with 2.4 mm titanium low-contact dynamic compression plates (Synthes USA, Paoli, PA). (*Courtesy of* Shriners Hospital for Children, Philadelphia, PA; with permission.)

forearm for correction greater than 90 degrees (Figs. 12–14). For a one-bone forearm, we transpose the radius onto the ulna into the desired position of forearm rotation (Figs. 15 and 16).

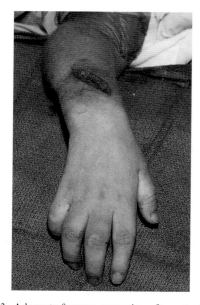

Fig. 13. Adequate forearm pronation after osteotomies of the radius and ulna. (*Courtesy of* Shriners Hospital for Children, Philadelphia, PA; with permission.)

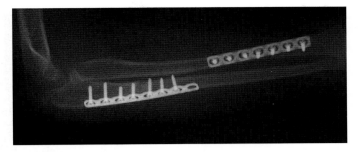

Fig. 14. Postoperative radiograph demonstrating union across osteotomies of the ulna and radius. (*Courtesy of* Shriners Hospital for Children, Philadelphia, PA; with permission.)

Children with intact extensor digitorum function (C7) and absent finger flexion (C8) are prone to develop MCP joint extension deformities (Fig. 17). Prophylactic night-time splinting in an intrinsic minus position will prevent the development of these contractures (Fig. 18). Because the hands of infants and toddlers are too small to benefit from commercially available splints, custom-made splints are required. This problem epitomizes the adage that "an ounce of prevention is worth a pound of cure." A fixed deformity impairs hand function, complicates surgical reconstruction, and is difficult to correct. Release of the MCP joint often results in less correction than expected and is prone to recurrence. Restoration of "balance" about the MCP joint is complicated. The absence of the primary MCP flexor (ie, the intrinsic muscles), the mediocre ability of the extrinsic flexors to flex the MCP joint, and the lack of donors for intrinsic transfer are all confounding factors. In children with active flexor digitorum superficialis and flexor digitorum profundus tendons, transfer of the superficialis tendons to the proximal phalanx rebalances the MCP joint and improves hand function.

Rehabilitation difficulties

Rehabilitation issues are complex and begin as soon as the cast is removed. We have developed a layman grading scale of tendon size to facilitate communication between the physician and therapist (Table 4). This scale gauges the strength of the tendon weave and guides the progression of therapy. Robust "linguine" tendons can be mobilized quickly without concern for disruption. In contrast, small "vermicelli" tendons require longer mobilization, prolonged splinting, increased protection, and a slower rehabilitation.

Similar techniques to learn tendon transfer apply to children and adults; however, the therapist must be adept with children and skilled at the techniques to mobilize tendon transfers. Active motion is crucial to prevent tendon scarring and facilitate muscle re-education; however, force must be limited, especially in children with small vermicelli tendons. The therapist must achieve the correct balance between motion and tendon protection. This principle requires expertise and is best performed by facilitates comfortable with pediatric tendon transfers. In addition, ongoing physician-therapist communication and inherent trust between the physician and therapist are mandatory items to achieve success.

Outcome

The principles and results of procedures for upper extremity reconstruction in adult SCI [24–27] are also applicable to children [28–30].

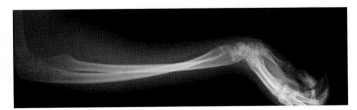

Fig. 15. Lateral radiograph of 100-degree fixed supination and excessive bowing of the ulna. (*Courtesy of* Shriners Hospital for Children, Philadelphia, PA; with permission.)

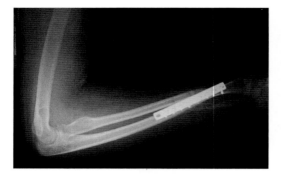

Fig. 16. Radiograph after transposition of the distal radius onto the proximal ulna to form a one-bone forearm. (*Courtesy of* Shriners Hospital for Children, Philadelphia, PA; with permission.)

Although the outcomes of tendon transfers on strength, excursion, and hand grasp and release abilities have been addressed in the literature, the outcomes on function and participation are only recently becoming clear. For children with C5 level SCI, tendon transfers and upper limb functional electrical stimulation increase independence by reducing the amount and level of support required by a personal care attendant. In addition, the ability to perform more activities is achieved. Despite these promising outcomes, children with C5 level SCI remain obligatory two-handed persons, even with tendon transfers and functional electrical stimulation. In contrast, through tendon transfers or functional electrical stimulation, children with C6 level SCI gain unilateral and bimanual function. For these children,

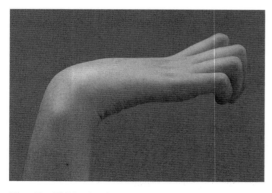

Fig. 17. Child who has C7 level SCI, intact extensor digitorum function, and absent finger flexion resulting in MCP joint extension deformities. (*Courtesy of* Shriners Hospital for Children, Philadelphia, PA; with permission.)

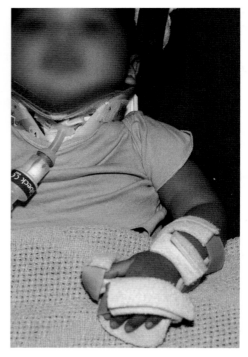

Fig. 18. Infant fitted with custom-made splint in an intrinsic minus position to prevent MCP joint extension deformities and the development of contractures. (*Courtesy of* Shriners Hospital for Children, Philadelphia, PA; with permission.)

upper limb reconstruction reduces or eliminates the need for adaptive equipment, enabling them to become more spontaneous throughout the day and exert less effort to complete a task. Because of these results and the importance of hand function for self-care, school, and play activities, we encourage children injured as infants and toddlers to undergo upper limb reconstruction as

Table 4
Grading scale of tendon size

Grade	Inference
Linguine	Early rehabilitation
	Little concern for repair failure
	Active motion to prevent motion limited scar
Spaghetti	Intermediate rehabilitation
Vermicelli or angel hair	Delayed rehabilitation
	Considerable concern for repair or failure
	Prolonged splint protection

soon as they are deemed candidates for the surgery and subsequent rehabilitation.

References

[1] Vogel LC, DeVivo MJ. Etiology and demographics. In: Betz RR, Mulcahey MJ, editors. The child with a spinal cord injury. Rosemont (IL): American Academy of Orthopaedic Surgeons; 1996. p. 3–12.

[2] Vogel LC, Anderson CJ. Spinal cord injuries in children and adolescents: a review. J Spinal Cord Med 2003;26:193–203.

[3] Vogel LC, DeVivo MJ. Pediatric spinal cord injury issues: etiology, demographics, and pathophysiology. Top Spinal Cord Inj Rehabil 1997;3:1–8.

[4] Betz RR, Mulcahey MJ, editors. The child with spinal cord injury. Rosemont (IL): American Academy of Orthopaedic Surgeons; 1996.

[5] Piatt JH, Steinberg M. Isolated spinal cord injury as a presentation of child abuse. Pediatrics 1995;96: 780–2.

[6] Feldman KW, Weinberger E, Milstein JM, et al. Cervical spine MRI in abused infants. Child Abuse Negl 1997;21:199–205.

[7] Shannon P, Smith CR, Deck J, et al. Axonal injury and the neuropathology of shaken baby syndrome. Neuropathology 1998;95:625–31.

[8] Dunne K, Hopkins IJ, Shield LK. Acute transverse myelopathy in childhood. Dev Med Child Neurol 1986;28:198–204.

[9] Knebusch M, Strassburg HM, Reiners K. Acute transverse myelitis in childhood: nine cases and review of the literature. Dev Med Child Neurol 1998;40:631–9.

[10] Ward WT. Atlanto-axial instability in children with Down syndrome. In: Betz RR, Mulcahey MJ, editors. The child with a spinal cord injury. Rosemont (IL): American Academy of Orthopaedic Surgeons; 1996. p. 89–96.

[11] Pang D, Wilberger JE. Spinal cord injury without radiographic abnormalities in children. J Neurosurg 1982;57:114–29.

[12] Mulcahey MJ. An overview of the upper extremity in pediatric spinal cord injury. Top Spinal Cord Inj Rehabil 1997;3(2):48–55.

[13] Clarkson HM, Gilewich GB. Musculoskeletal assessment: joint range of motion and manual muscle strength. Baltimore (MD): Williams & Wilkins; 1988. p. 20–6.

[14] Hislop H. Daniels and Worthingham's muscle testing: techniques of manual examination. Philadelphia: WB Saunders; 2002.

[15] McDowell CL, Moberg EA, House JH. The second international conference on surgical rehabilitation of the upper limb in tetraplegia (quadriplegia). J Hand Surg [Am] 1986;11:604–8.

[16] Kozin SH. Tetraplegia. Journal American Society for Surgery of the Hand 2002;2:141–52.

[17] Peckham PH, Kilgore KL, Keith MW, et al. An advanced neuroprosthesis for restoration of hand and upper arm control using an implantable controller. J Hand Surg [Am] 2002;27:265–76.

[18] Peckham PH, Gorman P. Functional electrical stimulation in the 21st century. Top Spinal Cord Inj Rehabil 2004;10:126–50.

[19] Paul SD, Gellman H, Waters R, et al. Single-stage reconstruction of key pinch and extension of the elbow in tetraplegic patients. J Bone Joint Surg [Am] 1994;76:1451–6.

[20] McGinley JC, Kozin SH. Interosseous membrane anatomy and functional mechanics. Clin Orthop 2001;383:108–22.

[21] Hankins SM, Bezwada HP, Kozin SH. Corrective osteotomies of the radius and ulna for supination contracture of the pediatric and adolescent forearm secondary to neurologic injury. J Hand Surg 2006; 31A:118–24.

[22] Zancolli EA. Paralytic supination contracture of the forearm. J Bone Joint Surg 1967;49A: 1275–84.

[23] Wang AA, Hutchinson DT, Coleman DA. One-bone forearm fusion for pediatric supination contracture due to neurologic deficit. J Hand Surg 2001;26A:611–6.

[24] Moberg E. Surgical rehabilitation of the upper limb in tetraplegia. Paraplegia 1990;2(8):330–4.

[25] Freehafer AA. Tendon transfers in patients with cervical spinal cord injury. J Hand Surg 1991;16A: 804–9.

[26] Zancolli E. Functional restoration of the upper limbs in traumatic quadriplegia. In: Zancolli E, editor. Structural and dynamic bases of hand surgery. 2nd edition. Philadelphia: Lippincott; 1979. p. 229–62.

[27] Mohammed K, Rothwell A, Sinclair S. Upper limb surgery for tetraplegia. J Bone Joint Surg 1992; 74B:873–9.

[28] Mulcahey MJ, Betz RR, Smith BT, et al. A prospective evaluation of upper extremity tendon transfers in children with cervical spinal cord injuries. J Pediatr Orthop 1999;19(3):319–28.

[29] Mulcahey MJ, Smith BT, Betz RR, et al. Functional neuromuscular stimulations: outcomes in young people with tetraplegia. J Spinal Cord Med 1994; 17(1):20–35.

[30] Mulcahey MJ, Smith BT, Betz RR, et al. The outcomes of surgical tendon transfers and occupational therapy in a child with a spinal cord injury. Am J Occup Ther 1995;49(7):607–17.

Index

Note: Page numbers of article titles are in **boldface** type.

A

American Spinal Injury Association (ASIA),
  A lesion (complete tetraplegia), 177
  B lesion (incomplete tetraplegia), 177
  C and D lesions, decisions for surgery in,
    178–179
  C lesion (incomplete tetraplegia), 177
  classification of cervical spinal cord lesions,
    175, 177
    hand surgeon and, 175, 177
    in children, 205
  D lesion (incomplete tetraplegia), 177

Anesthetics, to control spasticity, 179

Anterior (cord) syndrome, 176, 177

Arthrodeses, in severe incomplete lesions of spinal
  cord, 184

B

Baclofen, to control spasticity, 179

Biceps to triceps transfer, for active elbow
  extension, 193–199
    and deltoid to triceps transfer, compared,
      193
    discussion of, 198–199
    operative indications for, 194
    outcome of, clinical, 196–197
      dynamic EMG analysis of, 197–198
    prerequisite for, 209
    rehabilitation following, 195–196
    surgical technique for, 194–195, 196

Botulinum toxin (Botox), to control spasticity,
  180, 181

Brachial diplegia, 176

Brachioradialis to flexor pollicis longus transfer,
  for pinch reconstruction, 208

Brown-Sequard syndrome, 176–177

C

Central (cord) syndrome, 176, 178

Children, spinal cord injury in. See *Spinal cord,
  injury of, pediatric.*

D

Deltoid muscle, testing strength of, 186

Deltoid to triceps transfer, for active elbow
  extension, and biceps to triceps transfer,
  compared, 193
    discussion of, 192–193
    indication and contraindications to, 186
    outcome of, authors' series, 189–190, 191
      other series, 190–192
    polyaxial brace following, 189, 190
    postoperative regimen in, 189, 190
    surgical technique for, 187–189

Digitorum superficialis intrinsic transfer, for
  intrinsic function in hand reconstruction, 208

E

Elbow, active extension of, advantages
  of, 185–186
    surgical techniques for restoring, 186–199
  dysfunctional flexion contracture of, 185
  extension of, and wheelchair use, 211, 212
    reconstruction of, **185–201**
  full passive extension of, for pressure relief, 185

Elbow extension transfers, in management of
  upper limb in tetraplegia, 159

F

Finger and thumb extension, in hand
  reconstruction, 207

Forearm, fixed supination deformity of, 209
  one-bone, for forearm rotation, 210–211, 212

0749-0712/08/$ - see front matter © 2008 Elsevier Inc. All rights reserved.
doi:10.1016/S0749-0712(08)00044-9

hand.theclinics.com

Forearm (*continued*)
  passive rotation of, biceps re-routing for,
    209–210
  repositioning of, osteotomies of radius and
    ulna for, 210, 211
  surgical methods for, 210–211

G

Grasp, release, and pinch, reconstruction of, in
  management of upper limb in tetraplegia, 159
  tendon transfer for restoration of, 207

H

Hand, ability to use, versus activities-of-daily-
    living functioning, 164
  reconstruction of, finger and thumb extension
    in, 207
    intrinsic function in, digitorum superficialis
      intrinsic transfer for, 208

Hand surgeon, classification of cervical spinal
    cord lesions and, 177
  knowledge of patient's ASIA classification, 177
  reconstructive procedures in tetraplegia and,
    171

Hypertonicity/spasticity, of upper limbs, in
  incomplete lesions of spinal cord, 177–178

I

International Classification for Surgery of Hand
    in Tetraplegia (ICSHT), 169, 170, 205
  surgical guidelines based on, 205, 206

International Classification of Functioning
    Disability and Health (ICF), 161, 162
  as classification system, 165
  measurement tools and, 162

M

Metacarpophalangeal joint, extension deformities
    of, splinting in, 211, 212

Muscles, of upper limb, 175

N

Nerve blocks, peripheral, to control spasticity, 179

Neurectomy, total or partial, to control spasticity,
    180

O

Orthotics, in management of upper limb in
    tetraplegia, 159

Osteotomies, of radius and ulna, to reposition
    forearm, 210, 211

Outcomes measures, of management of upper
    limb in tetraplegia, 159, 163

P

Pinch, lateral, tendon transfer for restoration of,
    207
  reconstructiion of, in management of upper
    limb in tetraplegia, 159
  reconstruction of, brachioradialis to flexor
    pollicis longus transfer for, 208

R

Radius and ulna, osteotomies of, to reposition
    forearm, 210, 211

S

Spasticity, control of, in severe incomplete spinal
    cord lesions, 179–180

Spinal cord, cervical, complete lesion of, surgical
    rehabilitation in, 178
  incomplete lesions of, 175–176
    management of upper limb in, **175–184**
    painful contractures in, 178
    painful hyperesthesias in, 178
    severe, arthrodeses in, 184
      control of spasticity in, 179–180
      tendon transfers in, 180–182
      tenodeses in, 184
      tenotomies/muscle-tendon
        lengthening and capsulotomies in,
        182–183
    surgical decisions in, 178–179
    upper limb evaluation in, 177–178
    upper limb hypertonicity/spasticity in,
      177–178
  incomplete transection of, 176
  injury(ies) of, clinical syndromes of,
    176–177
    systems of injury classifications and, 175
  paralyzed upper extremity muscles with
    distal muscle sparing in, 178
  injury of, pediatric, initial evaluation in,
    203–204
    life expectancy in, 203
    management of upper limb tetraplegia
      in, **203–213**
    mechanisms of, 203
    preoperative considerations in, 204–206
    surgery in, age at, 204

approach for, 206–208
    assessment for, 205–206
    obstacles to, 208–211
    outcome of, 211–212
    rehabilitation following, 211

Splinting, in metacarpophalangeal joint extension
    deformities, 211, 212

T

Tendon transfer(s), grasp restoration following,
    207
    in severe incomplete spinal cord lesions,
        180–182
    lateral pinch restoration following, 207

Tenodeses, in severe incomplete lesions of spinal
    cord, 184

Tenotomies/muscle-tendon lengthening and
    capsulotomies, in severe incomplete spinal
    cord lesions, 182–183

Tetraplegia, assessment of, outcome measures
        and, 163
    timed testing and, 164
    at level of C5, C6, or C7, movement below
        elbow and, 162
    conservative treatment in, 162
    measurement issues in, 163–165
        and contextual factors, 164
        physiologic evaluation and, 163–164
    measurement of, timing of, 164–165
    motor skill acquisition, and learning process
        of, 166
    outcomes of interest in, 165
    reach in, wheelchair use and, 185
    reconstructive procedures in, hand surgeons
        and, 171
        influence of cost and coverage of on, 172
        negative attitudes of patients and, 172
        results of, 171
        spinal cord specialists and surgeons in, 171

underutilization of, 169–172
reconstructive upper limb surgery in,
    classification of, 169
    current utilization of, **169–173**
    evaluation for, 169
    timing of measurement in, 164–165
upper limb in, management of, Asian data
        sources on, 158
        contemporary trends in, **157–160**
        elbow extension transfers and, 159
        European data sources on, 158
        grasp, release, and pinch in, 159
        in pediatric spinal cord injury, **203–213**
        incomplete lesions and, 159
        methods and materials for, 157
        orthotics and, 159
        outcomes measures and, 160
        referral to hand program and, 159
        solicited data points on, 158
upper limb interventions in, measurement
        issues related to, **161–168**
    outcomes in, measurement of, 162
    timed testing of, 164
weakness of patients with, 172

U

Upper limbs, evaluation of, in incomplete lesions
    of spinal cord, 177–178
    hypertonicity/spasticity in, in incomplete
        lesions of spinal cord, 177–178
    in tetraplegia. See *Tetraplegia, upper limb in.*
    key muscles of, 175
    management of, in incomplete lesions of
        cervical spinal cord, **175–184**
    reconstructive surgery in, in tetraplegia,
        current utilization in, **169–173**

W

Wheelchair use, reach of tetraplegic patient and,
    185